Semaglutides

ONCE A WEEK
WEIGHT LOSS
INJECTIONS

Semaglutides

ONCE A WEEK
WEIGHT LOSS
INJECTIONS

- Zepbound
- Wegovy
- Ozempic
- Mounjaro

RICHARD L.
LIPMAN M.D.

Book Cover Design: David Colon
Book Formatting: Creative Publishing Book Design

Table of Contents

Disclaimer

The reading of this book does not establish a doctor-patient relationship between the reader and Dr Lipman. As discussed numerous times in this book, successful weight loss requires a personal relationship with an understanding physician.

This book does not substitute for professional or medical advice. The author and the publisher specifically disclaim any liability, loss, or risk, personal or otherwise that might be incurred, directly or indirectly, as a result of the use and application of any of the contents of this book. All matters regarding your health require a physician's medical consultation and supervision. The names and identifying characteristics of the individuals referred to in anecdotes within this book have been changed to protect their identities.

www.richardlipmanmd.com

Acknowledgments

I would like to thank the thousands and thousands of patients I have treated over the years who inspired me to discover new methods to treat some of the simplest problems we all have. To my brothers, David and Sidney, my oldest friends and supporters who have always been there in times of peril and joy. To my grandchildren, Chelsea, Jason, Jessica, Samantha and Savannah, you remain my most devoted followers, and to my children Jeffrey, David, Missy and Andrea, we made it! To my wife of 48 years, Jacqueline, you will always be my inspiration and love of my life.

Writing a book is harder than I thought and more rewarding than I could have ever imagined. Special thanks to my long time assistant Claudia Morales for her support and kind suggestions. I am grateful to my book editor Chidinma Dinwoke from Nigeria who never failed to respond to my many changes, David Colon from Spain for a great book cover and Julian Thomas from Romania for his incredible graphics. Without your help, I would never have completed this book.

Drug Nomenclature Update

Two closely related groups of medications are discussed in this book. Semaglutides (Ozempic and Wegovy) belong to a class of medications known as glucagon-like peptide-1 (GLP-1) receptor agonists. They mimic the GLP-1 hormone that is released in the gastrointestinal tract in response to eating. Ozempic has FDA approval for the treatment of diabetes while Wegovy is FDA approved for weight loss. They are identical medications.

The second group of drugs are termed Tirzepatides (Mounjaro and Zepbound). Tirzepatides are in a class of medications called glucose-dependent insulinotropic polypeptide (GIP) receptor **and** glucagon-like peptide-1 (GLP-1) receptor agonists. Mounjaro has FDA approval for diabetes while Zepbound (approved in November 2023) is approved for weight loss. Mounjaro and Zepbound are identical drugs.

Since both group of medications contain GLP-1 receptor agonists they are often grouped together as Semagludies, although the Tirzepatides do have a second peptide with slightly different actions.

CHAPTER 1

Introducing the Semaglutide Weight Loss Plan

Welcome to "Semaglutides: Once a Week Weight Loss Injections" your guide to unlocking the transformative power of the Semaglutides: Ozempic, Wegovy and the Tirzepatides Zepbound and Mounjaro. This group of medications not only provides rapid and safe weight loss, reduces comorbidities such as hypertension, diabetes and elevated cholesterol, and also offers long-term weight loss maintenance. Whether you're tired of yo-yo dieting or looking for a fresh approach to shedding those stubborn pounds, Semaglutide, including medications like Ozempic, Wegovy, Zepbound and Mounjaro, add an exciting new frontier in weight management.

In recent years, the world has witnessed a staggering rise in obesity rates with three out of four Americans overweight or obese. This has lead to a host of health complications and diminished quality of life for countless individuals. Life style changes such as adhering to a rigorous diet and engaging in strenuous physical activity are insufficient not only for sustaining weight loss but for reversing the comorbidities of obesity.

Pharmacological methods for weight loss are becoming an increasingly important therapeutic option. However, despite the vast number of overweight and obese people, few even consider medications. Some of this hesitation may be attributed to the fact that older weight loss medications fail to result in weight reduction of more than five to six percent, have numerous undesirable side effects and are unable to result in long term weight loss maintenance.

Semaglutide Group of Medications Offer New Hopes for Obesity Treatment

Recognizing this pressing need, medical science has made significant strides to develop innovative treatments that address the weight loss challenges effectively. Semaglutides including Ozempic and Wegovy, glucagon-like peptide-1 (GLP-1) receptor agonists, and more recently the newly approved Tirzepatides Zepbound and Mounjaro have emerged as game-changers in this arena.

All four medications mimic the naturally occurring hormone called glucagon-like peptide 1 or simply GLP-1. They control insulin and glucagon secretion resulting in control of blood sugar food intake and cravings. Long-acting versions of other GLP-1 receptor agonists have been on the market for over a decade such as Liraglutide (Victoza, Saxenda), Dulaglutide (Trulicity) and Exenatide (Byetta, Bydureon). The newer versions marketed as Ozempic and Wegovy are considered among the most powerful weight loss medications. Zepbound and Mounjaro were recently released that have a second peptide termed glucose-dependent insulinotropic polypeptide or GIP added to the GLP-1 agonist. A fourth Semaglutide, Retatrutide containing three peptides, with reported average weight loss of 27%, is currently in stage 3 Clinical Trials.

Since the two medications are very similar in action and side effects, I have called them all "Semaglutides" and only refer to Tirzepatide when there are specific differences.

Semaglutide Medications Have Impact All Over the Body

Unlike the older weight loss medications, Semaglutide medications act specifically on receptors in the brain's appetite and reward centers, the pancreas, muscle, liver, and even the stomach. The result is a marked decrease in appetite, cravings, hunger, and a delay in gastric emptying. The latter effect produces prolonged satiety and fullness. As a result, the body is taking in fewer calories, resulting in progressive weight loss that often starts soon after beginning therapy. *Semaglutides do not have side effects of anxiety, depression, insomnia, palpitations, and a racy heart, as seen with the older diet medications.*

Weight Loss and Beyond: Semaglutide Treatment

Traditionally, obesity therapy has centered on lifestyle modifications including elaborate diets to restrict food intake, counting grams of protein, carbs or fat and exercise to enhance metabolism. Regrettably, we are recognizing that the body uses a variety of counter-regulatory processes to hinder weight reduction by decreasing metabolism and increasing cravings during and after weight loss to promote eating and subsequent weight gain.

I have personally treated hundreds of overweight and obese people with these medications. Weight loss of 25-30% of starting weight is common because of the drugs' effect on appetite, fullness, cravings, and metabolism. Even after only a few days of therapy, some of my patients tell me their cravings for sweets, fatty food, and alcohol have disappeared. This often happens before they notice weight loss. Uniformly they say that they have much less compulsion to eat. Social media calls it "Food Noise" which is a colloquial term referring to constant thoughts or recurring ruminations about food.

In addition to weight loss and elimination of cravings, Semaglutide therapy is associated with improvements in blood sugar in people with diabetes, reduction of blood pressure and cholesterol levels, and improvement in other cardiovascular markers.

Semaglutides' exceptional success is due, in part, to their action in multiple organs, the absence of tachyphylaxis (drug tolerance), which is present in practically all other weight loss drugs, the lack of significant side effects as well as the amazing effect on appetite, cravings, and fullness. The Semaglutides have been designed to be taken indefinitely, like any other medication for a chronic problem.

There are several reasons why healthcare professionals treat relatively few patients with anti-obesity drugs. This includes not only the unwillingness of public health and medical organizations to recognize obesity as a disease but also the lack of insurance reimbursement. Making matters worse is the belief that most obese individuals are unable to lose weight and, more importantly, keep it off because they lack willpower.

Overweight and Obese Individuals Have Altered Brain Chemistry Making It Difficult to Lose Weight and Keep It Off

We now know that, through no fault of their own, the brains of overweight and obese individuals vary biochemically from those of normal weight people. Even after losing significant weight, obese people lack the natural physiological and hormonal cues to stop overeating. They are either deficient in hormones and chemicals or do not respond correctly to those chemicals. As a result, they eat the incorrect foods or consume excessive amounts of food.

Mild Side Effects Found with Semaglutides Usually Disappear with Treatment

Side effects reported in clinical testing of these medications involve mainly the gastrointestinal tract and range from mild to moderate that are tolerable and disappear as the drugs are taken. Supporting the observations of only very mild side effects is the fact that only 7% of subjects in one large study withdrew from Semaglutide treatment because of adverse reactions. My experience is even more amazing, only 3-4 % of patients have needed to stop semaglutides due to adverse effects.

The Semaglutide Food Plan is Simple and Easy to Remember

This new weight loss plan is based on a simple food plan that minimizes carbs and maximizes proteins. There are no problematic culinary preparations. There is no shopping for uncommon foods, or counting calories, carbohydrates, fat, protein, or anything else. There are no recipes at all! Understanding what makes you hungry and what makes you full will allow you to eat normally and remove most of your hunger and cravings even before you start taking the medication.

Weight Maintenance: The Core of the Semaglutide Plan

In the Semaglutide Plan, the emphasis is on weight maintenance from the first day of therapy. This involves first identifying the most significant causes of weight gain, discovering reduced calorie and carb substitutes and then determining the best Semaglutide medication for weight loss and maintenance. Unfortunately, this is often based on insurance coverage, availability, and cost.

Semaglutide maintenance begins once the patient has reached his/her goal and consists of increasing the daily caloric intake, tapering the Semaglutide injection frequency and dose and adopting a workable exercise plan.

You and your doctor will discover a long-term solution to losing and maintaining weight. It is never a matter of special recipes, counting anything or hoping to use willpower alone. It is about limiting hunger and cravings using your body's natural hormones and taking one of the Semaglutide injections first weekly to lose the weight then on a longer term basis once or twice a month to maintain the weight loss.

For the millions of overweight people who have or are at high risk of developing medical issues due to their weight, particularly hypertension and type 2 diabetes, Zepbound, Mounjaro, Ozempic, and Wegovy will be their best choice. These medications, in combination with the reduced calorie, and low-carb diet outlined here, will assist patients in achieving and maintaining their targeted weight loss.

Semaglutide Weight Loss: FAQs

The *Semaglutide Weight Loss Plan* is based on 4 new FDA-approved prescription medications which include Ozempic, Wegovy, Zepbound and Mounjaro. Since they are very similar, they are grouped together under "Semaglutides."

Ozempic was approved (2018) for diabetes; *Wegovy*, a higher dose of Ozempic was approved (2021) for weight loss; and *Mounjaro* was approved (2022) for diabetes. Mounjaro is used "off label" pending FDA approval as an obesity drug. This occurred in November 2023 with the name change to Zepbound. A reduced-calorie, high-protein, low-carb food plan has been added to increase the weight loss. Ozempic and Wegovy consist of a single hormone, GLP-1 while Tirzepatides have a second hormone, GIP. The following are common FAQs associated with the use of Semaglutides.

How Do The Semaglutides Work?

They act specifically on receptors in the brain's appetite centers, the pancreas, muscle, liver, by decreasing appetite, cravings, hunger, and delaying gastric emptying. As a result, the body takes in fewer calories, resulting in progressive weight loss that often starts after a few days of therapy.

What are Adverse Reactions of Semaglutides?

Adverse reactions and side effects are almost all gastrointestinal including nausea, vomiting, constipation and abdominal pain. Gall bladder problems, fatigue, and mild hypoglycemic reactions occur rarely. *Semaglutides are variations in normal hormones and do not cause anxiety, depression, insomnia, palpitations, rises in blood pressure, and a racy heart, as with the older diet medications.*

Do Semaglutides Interact with other Medications or other Medical Problems?

Not significant. Because Semaglutides have almost identical structures as normally occurring hormones, no interactions with other drugs or other medical problems such as thyroid, cardiac or pulmonary diseases have been reported.

Which Semaglutide is Best for Weight Loss?

Not Much Difference. All have similar ingredients and side effects—nausea, constipation, diarrhea, abdominal pain, rare vomiting. Zepbound and Mounjaro might be slightly more effective because they have a second hormone as an ingredient. These drugs are expensive, have limited availability, and poor insurance coverage.

Do I Need to Change My Diet to Lose Weight?

Of Course, You Do! You cannot lose weight drinking high-sugar beverages, too much alcohol, fast foods, pastries, rice, pasta, and potatoes very often. Dr. Lipman's Semaglutide Food Plan offers a simple, low-carb food plan that is used with these medications. Weight loss is easy following the Rules of Ten from Dr Lipman's Food Plan.

Do I Need Any Tests Before Taking these Medications?

The common metabolic tests such as a chemistry profile, thyroid tests, A1C (test for diabetes), blood count, and cholesterol are suggested. Recent tests (less than 3 months ago) may be acceptable. If using a virtual visit, a blood pressure reading and weight are *always* required.

How are the Medications Taken?

Self-injected using a pen injector just under the skin in the abdomen *once* a week (usually on Friday or Saturday). The few oral versions are not very effective. The doses start low and are gradually increased, if needed.

How Much Weight Can I Expect to Lose?

Studies show an average weight loss of 15 to 25 % of starting weight. Weight loss starts 5-10 days after the first injection. It's not unusual to see 10 to 15 lb. weight loss in the first month.

What is the Starting Dose of these Medications?

Start with the lowest doses of 0.25 or 0.5 mg per week of Ozempic, Wegovy or 2.5 or 5 mg per week of Zepbound and Mounjaro and increase monthly, if needed depending on the amount of weight loss and the side effects.

What is the Cost of the Semaglutide Injections?

These drugs are expensive. Costs vary by pharmacy. Use www.goodrx.com to check current costs and obtain a savings coupon that is good at most pharmacies.

Will the Cravings be Controlled?

Cravings for sweets, salty food and alcohol are markedly decreased in a few days in some people and by ten days in the remainder. "Food noise"-the constant preoccupation with eating is remarkably eliminated in almost all people taking these medications, often within a few days of starting the program.

What Causes Slow Weight Loss with Semaglutides?

Slow weight loss can be due to low starting weight, age, gender, and medical problems (like diabetes or low thyroid) as well as medications you might be taking for other problems. Other causes of slow weight loss are lowering of metabolism with weight loss and even errors in the diet plan such as drinking too many carbonated beverages, and skipping meals.

What are the Benefits of Semaglutides?

Semaglutides produce rapid weight loss by marked reduction in caloric intake. This is associated with improvement in comorbidities including high blood pressure, elevated blood sugar, high cholesterol, sleep apnea and arthritis. Recent reports show that fatty liver from obesity can be reversed with these medications. Compulsive eating, often call "food noise" is remarkably reduced.

How do I Maintain the Weight Loss?

Dr Lipman's plan for weight maintenance is based on continuing the Semaglutide injections at a lower dose and frequency and following the principles of his food plan.

What Do I Do When I Reach My Goal Weight?

The prospect of regaining the weight after weight loss is very high (maybe 80%), despite the best intentions including daily exercise and careful food intake. The intense hormonal factors that produce this weight rebound can result in a slow rise in blood sugar, blood pressure, arthritis, and sleep apnea in individuals that experienced these problems before the weight loss. The consensus is that the Semaglutide injections should be continued for a long period. Dr. Lipman believes the frequency or dose can be lowered to twice a month.

Side Effects, Adverse Effects and Warnings

- *Pancreatitis:* Has been reported in clinical trials. But very rare. Discontinue promptly if pancreatitis is suspected.
- *Hypoglycemia with Concomitant Use of Insulin Secretagogues or Insulin*
- *Hypersensitivity Reactions:* Hypersensitivity reactions have been reported. Discontinue if suspected. Local injection site reactions can be treated with Bendryl 25 mg OTC and/or OTC steroid creams.
- *Mild to Moderate Gastrointestinal Disease:* Use may be associated with gastrointestinal adverse reactions.
- *Acute Gallbladder Disease:* Has occurred rarely in clinical trials.

Most Common Adverse Effects

Reported in ≥5% of patients treated are: nausea, diarrhea, vomiting, constipation, dyspepsia, and abdominal pain. Nausea is easily treated with Zofran, dyspepsia and abdominal pain with Prilosec, Pepcid or Tagment.

Who Can Be Prescribed These Medications?

The decision to start taking a weight loss medication is a personal one. If diet and exercise changes aren't enough, you and your healthcare provider may consider weight loss medications, if you have: a body mass index (BMI) greater than 30 or a BMI of 27 or more with other related health problems, such as hypertension, high cholesterol, heart disease, or diabetes.

Who Should NOT Take These Medications?

(https://uspl.lilly.com/mounjaro/) (https://www.novo-pi.com/wegovy/) Personal or family history of medullary thyroid carcinoma or in patients with Multiple Endocrine Neoplasia Syndrome type 2, known serious hypersensitivity to Semaglutide or Tirzepatide.

Pregnancy: Based on animal studies, Semaglutides may cause fetal harm, and breastfeeding.

CC, a recent patient of mine told me that he had struggled with his weight all his life. After losing 6 lb. in a week, he said to me, "No wonder skinny people think heavy people have no willpower. Their brains actually do tell them to stop eating. I had no idea."

MR has told me for 20 years that her whole day revolves around thinking about food. I never really understood it until she told me about her experience with Ozempic. Before Ozempic, when she woke up she was not only thinking about breakfast but also about what she was going to have for lunch. As soon as she had lunch, she was thinking about dinner. Driving home after work at 3 pm, she would stop at Dunkin Donuts for her favorite, Chocolate Frosted Donut with Sprinkles. She said there was always chatter in her head about food. Three days after starting the Ozempic she called and told me "it's the strangest thing; I don't have any cravings any more—it's like someone turned off a switch in my head."

CHAPTER 2

Do You Have Metabolic Syndrome?

Metabolic Syndrome is a group of abnormal metabolic changes that have become more common as Americans gained weight during the past 15 years. These abnormalities include an accumulation of fat in and around the abdomen, high blood pressure, and diabetes, high cholesterol, increased risk of heart disease, and elevated triglycerides (fats) in the blood.

All these abnormalities result from the excess food we consume turning to fat which is first stored around the belly. After accumulating on the outside of the belly, that common "beer belly" fat is stored inside the abdomen around the internal organs. Figure 2.1 illustrates a whole family with metabolic syndrome.

Figure 2.1: *This Whole Family Has the Metabolic Syndrome*

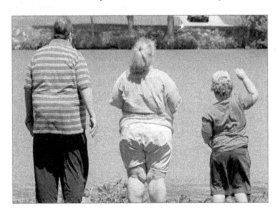

These new fat cells around and inside the abdomen synthesize new chemicals not present before the weight gain. The chemicals leave the fat cells and travel via the bloodstream all over the body, causing widespread inflammation, raising blood pressure and injuring the heart and blood vessels. The result is hypertension, diabetes, heart attacks, and strokes—the signs of Metabolic Syndrome.

Metabolic Syndrome affects most patients who have gained 30 pounds or more. They are typically unaware of the problem when they initially enter my office. They are surprised to learn that the fat cells around and inside their belly (often a subject of ridicule) convert into an active brand-new endocrine organ like the thyroid or adrenal gland, producing a slew of harmful new chemicals that are released into the bloodstream.

The hallmark of Metabolic Syndrome is too much fat around the abdomen. It is the cause of the disease. You do not need an expensive blood test, an MRI, or to see a doctor to confirm that you have it.

If you are a woman with a waistline of 35 inches or more or man with a waistline of 40 inches or more, you are well on your way to Metabolic Syndrome.

In figure 2.2, enlarging fat cells are deposited around intra-abdominal organs, the hallmark of the metabolic syndrome. The fat cells are indicated in yellow and are divided into two types. Extra-abdominal fat is the fat below the skin (A) and visceral fat is inside the abdomen, labeled B. It's the visceral fat that causes all of the medical problems of obesity.

According to current data, more than 35% of the population today has Metabolic Syndrome. Some doctors believe that if obesity continues to increase at the current rate, 85 %–92 % of Americans will have Metabolic Syndrome by 2035.

Figure 2.2: *Fat Cells Surround the Intra-Abdominal Organs in Metabolic Syndrome*

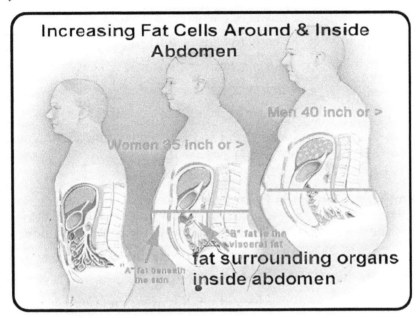

How is Metabolic Syndrome Discovered?

Since the first signs of metabolic Syndrome are mostly chemical changes in the blood, the first symptoms you might notice are delayed for years. Other than the warning of unusual weight gain and a protruding belly, there are no signs.

Metabolic Syndrome presents a fivefold increased risk of dying of cardiac disease in the ten years after diagnosis and a tenfold risk of developing diabetes.

What Causes the Metabolic Changes in the Blood in People with Metabolic Syndrome?

When we consume more food than we need for energy, excess food is converted into fat stored in fat cells scattered all over the body.

These fat deposits are normal and serve as an energy source when food is limited.

The problem begins when food intake continues to be in excess—above the amount the body recognizes as needed for "normal energy storage." When this happens, excess fat is stored in newly created fat cells around the waist and inside of the abdomen. These new fat cells are different from the older fat cells. They act like a filter removing chemicals from the bloodstream and at the same time releasing new proteins and chemicals into the bloodstream.

Enlarging Fat Cells Effect on Insulin

The enlarging fat cells deactivate insulin and cause a condition known as insulin resistance. The body makes insulin, but the fat cells render the insulin less effective in lowering blood sugar. This causes the pancreas to work harder and produce more and more insulin to control the blood sugar. When the pancreas cannot keep up with the increasing demand for insulin, the fasting blood sugar rises, and the person is said to have type 2 diabetes. It's all a vicious circle of increased sugar driving more and more insulin production that is relatively ineffective.

Diabetes in obese people is associated with *more* and *not less insulin*. The defect is that the enlarging abdominal fat cells have rendered the insulin less active and effective in controlling blood sugar. This explains the relationship between enlarging fat cells due to excess food ingestion and the development of overt diabetes.

Enlarging Fat Cells Produce New Chemicals

Enlarging fat cells inside and outside the belly produce ninety new chemicals including several hormones and multiple proteins that were *not* present before the excess weight gain. These substances function as chemical messengers between the fat cells and the rest of the body. They raise triglyceride levels, blood pressure, and blood sugar, cause blood clots and polycystic ovaries, as well as heart attacks and strokes.

Here are some of the key criteria (figure 2.3) for Metabolic Syndrome. Note: At first glance, the excess weight in an individual with Metabolic Syndrome is concentrated around the waist. This is called central obesity. It is the hallmark of Metabolic Syndrome. All the other criteria are metabolic abnormalities seen in the blood measurements.

Figure 2.3 *Metabolic Criteria for the Metabolic Syndrome*

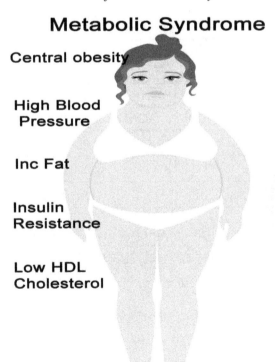

Metabolic Syndrome

Central obesity

High Blood Pressure

Inc Fat

Insulin Resistance

Low HDL Cholesterol

Five Criteria to Determine If You Have *Metabolic Syndrome*

1. Waist Circumference: 40 inches or more for men; 35 inches or more for women.

Forty inches and 35 inches are the average measurements. To be more accurate, you need to relate waist obesity with height. Here are the measurements based on size for both genders. Waist is measured at the top of the iliac crest using the National Institute of Health criteria.

The waist circumference as seen in Table 2.1 is the most reliable measurement for determination of the Metabolic Syndrome.

Table 2.1 *Waist Circumference Helps Define Metabolic Syndrome*

Criteria for Waist Circumference in Adults			
Waist Circumferences			
Risk Category	Females		Males	
	cm	in	cm	in
Very Low	<70	28.5	<80	31.5
Low	70-89	28.5-35.0	80-99	31.5-39.0
High	90-109	35.5-43.0	100-120	39.5-47.0
Very High	>109	>43.0	>120	>47.0

2. Blood pressure: 130/85 mmHg or higher

The ideal blood pressure is 120/70. The value of 130/85 is slightly elevated from the ideal.

3. Triglyceride: levels above 150 mg/ml

Triglycerides are the fat in the blood. They come from our food and are also produced by the liver and fat cells. As the level of triglycerides increases, fat and cholesterol are deposited as plaques which narrow the blood supply to arteries around the heart (coronary arteriosclerosis) and in the brain (cerebral arteriosclerosis). This results in possible angina (chest pain), heart attacks, and strokes.

4. Fasting blood sugar: values greater than 100 mg/ml or High A1C

Normal fasting blood sugar is from 70 to 99 mg/ml. When blood sugar rises above 100 mg, the pancreas (the organ responsible for insulin production) cannot keep up with the rising blood sugar. Although insulin levels are high, it's ineffective in lowering blood sugar. Diabetes is the result. An elevated A1C is a more accurate measurement of average blood sugar over the past three months.

Here are the A1C values from normal to diabetic:

- Normal A1C: 5.6% or less
- Pre-diabetic A1C: 5.7-6.3
- Diabetic A1C: 6.4 or >

5. HDL (good cholesterol): less than 50

Cholesterol is a fatty chemical made in the liver and in the fat cells of overweight people. The two main types are HDL or high-density cholesterol or "good cholesterol," and LDL cholesterol or low-density cholesterol (bad cholesterol). Figure 2.4 shows LDL cholesterol sticking to artery walls. This causes heart disease and strokes by the block of blood flow through the heart and blood vessels.

In Metabolic Syndrome, the HDL cholesterol is low, thus preventing the "cleaning "of the blood vessels. The "protective" effect of high HDL is absent in Metabolic Syndrome. A good number for HDL cholesterol is about 70 or 80. Exercise and dietary changes can raise it.

Figure 2.4 *Cholesterol Plaque Partially Blocking Blood Flow in Artery*

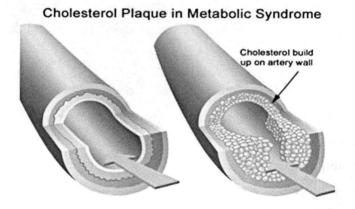

Body Mass Index and Obesity and Morbidity

Body mass index (BMI) is a medical screening technique that estimates the amount of body fat based on the weight-to-height ratio. BMI is determined by dividing weight in kilograms (kg) by square of the height in meters (m²). BMI is usually correlated with body fat—the higher the value, the more body fat. However, BMI is not a great metric because it does not examine body fat directly. Because muscle and bone are denser than fat, an athlete or muscular person might have a high BMI without being overweight. However, most individuals are not athletes, and BMI is a fairly accurate indicator of their percentage of body fat for most people.

Healthy BMI in Adults: The World Health Organization (WHO) states that for adults, the healthy range for BMI is between 18.5 and 24.9.

- *Overweight* is defined as a body mass index of 25 to 29.9.
- *Obesity is defined as a* body mass index of 30 or higher.

These BMI cut off points in adults are the same for men and women, regardless of their age. Table 2.2 provides a BMI table for adults.

Table 2.2. BMI Table *Standard BMI table Relates Weight to Height*

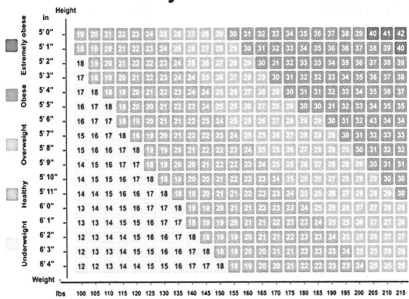

Metabolic Syndrome is a complex condition related to genetic factors and excess food intake. The capacity to reduce weight and boost energy production via exercise are important methods for dealing with the impacts of metabolic syndrome. The graph in Figure 2.5 shows the relationship between increasing weight gain

Figure 2.5 *BMI vs. Mortality Risk*

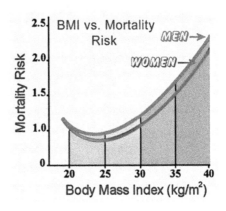

and mortality. For example, a woman with a BMI of 37 has a risk of dying which is two times the average. It's estimated that the mortality of individual with a BMI of 40 or more is the same as someone who smoked 2 packs of cigarettes for 30 years.

The use of Semaglutides can help achieve meaningful weight loss and often reverse the comorbidities of weight gain.

DC, an importer of rare plants in South Florida has Metabolic Syndrome with diabetes, hypertension, high cholesterol, and fatty liver as complications of his long-standing obesity. After taking 15 mg of Mounjaro for 4 months, his weight fell from 237 lb. to 176 lb., his blood sugar from 277 to 85, his A1C from 7.2 to 5.1, his AST (liver test) from 64 to 26. His sugar and alcohol cravings have disappeared.

CHAPTER 3

Internal and External Signals Tell Us to Eat or Not to Eat

When launching a weight loss program, it is important to initially deal with the two issues that are the largest hindrances to any sustainable diet: hunger and cravings. People will give up dieting solely to get rid of hunger and cravings. Hundreds of internal signals including multiple hormones and external stimuli bombard our brain with instructions telling us whether we should eat or not. And the messages always say, "Eat!"

Making matters worse, individuals who are trying to lose weight are frequently unable to distinguish between true hunger, cravings, low blood sugar, simple habit, and other signals such as exhaustion, stress, and boredom.

Hunger or Cravings: Which is It?

When we go several hours without eating, our natural reaction is to become hungry. It's our body's way of telling us we need to eat. Hunger is the rumbling of our bellies, which is accompanied by lethargy, weakness, and thoughts of food. Cravings are a strong, illogical desire for certain foods. Cravings can arise when we are not hungry. Hunger is a physiological need. Cravings are psychological impulses. Figure 3.1 presents a list of factors producing hunger.

Figure 3.1 *Multiple factors that can produce feelings of hunger*

> **Three Factors Can Produce Feelings of Hunger:**
>
> 1. Hormones in the blood and brain can produce feelings of hunger or fullness: Ghrelin and Leptin.
> 2. External cues and stimuli tell us to: "eat" or "not eat."
> 3. Certain foods tell us we are hungry or full.

Hormones Produce Fullness or Hunger: Leptin and Ghrelin

Two hormones are involved in appetite control—*Leptin* which is made in fat cells, and *Ghrelin* which is produced in the stomach. This is illustrated in figure 3.2. Both signal our appetite centers in opposite directions. Leptin tells our appetite centers that our fat cells are full and that there is *no need to eat* while Ghrelin tells our brain that the stomach is empty and that we *need to eat*.

Figure 3.2 *Leptin and Ghrelin Control Food Intake*

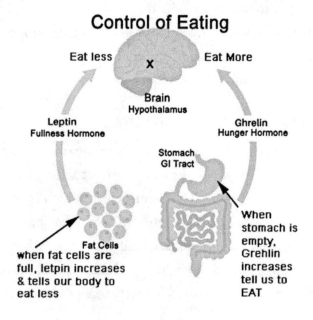

Control of Eating

Eat less — X — Eat More

Brain
Hypothalamus

Leptin
Fullness Hormone

Ghrelin
Hunger Hormone

Stomach
GI Tract

Fat Cells
when fat cells are full, letpin increases & tells our body to eat less

When stomach is empty, Grehlin increases tell us to EAT

It was first believed that overweight individuals might be overeating because they have too little leptin. But that is not the case. In fact, obese people have too much leptin. However, their brains do not recognize the leptin present and function as if there is no leptin at all. People in this category feel as though they are starving all the time, so they eat constantly. This process is similar to type 2 diabetes, where insulin levels are high, but insulin, just like leptin, simply becomes ineffective.

One of the major reasons that people regain their lost weight after a diet is that the body responds to the lost fat and muscle with an increase in Ghrelin and other appetite encouraging hormones

Hunger is Triggered by External Cues to Eat Even When Not Hungry

Hunger is influenced not just by chemicals in the brain, but also by a variety of external cues such on time of day, fatigue, habits, and even food and drinks seen on TV. Billboard signs and even the tiny video screens we see when pumping gas remind us that tasty snacks are only a few feet away. Smells and even sounds can often stimulate the desire to eat. Focusing on how exterior signals can establish hunger (or what is misunderstood as hunger) is extremely important since overweight people appear to overreact to these stimuli. The rapid rise in excess weight over the previous half-century is not attributable to any new changes in the body's hormones, but rather to increasingly prominent outside cues prompting our desire to eat.

Very few overweight individuals are hungry solely because of hormonal abnormalities. For most people, hunger is the result of hormonal abnormalities combined with powerful external signals. That is why willpower is ineffective and some weight regain follows almost all weight loss plans! Anyone attempting to lose weight must

25

first learn to protect him or herself from signals and cues that evoke hunger even when they are not hungry.

Emotional Cues and Signals That Tell Us to EAT or Not EAT

1. Stress: Stress is thought to be a major cause of overeating. The nature of the stress may play the most important role in overeating. Major stress causes less eating and minor stress may cause increased eating. Major stressors are less frequent in our lives than minor stressors, which is potentially a significant reason for the preponderance of overeating.

Overeating is affected by stress type and dietary preferences. High calorie sweet or salty snacks are preferred over meat, vegetables, and fruits. They seldom satisfy hunger and make you want more, regardless of physiological requirements. Stress-related eating causes long-term problems with weight control.

2. Fatigue: Some people cannot distinguish between hunger and fatigue. With fatigue, someone can be just as hungry after a large meal as they would be if they had not eaten for a whole day. A 1999 study at the University of Chicago found that sleeping only four hours a night for four days resulted in a decrease in metabolism and an increase in hunger.

3. Boredom, depression, and anxiety: These psychological problems are well-known causes of overeating. Food will not affect these conditions or change the situations that caused them. Yet people often find themselves looking for even more comfort food. What to do?

If it is depression and anxiety, you need to take care of your mental health first. A little physical exercise will make a real difference in how you feel.

4. Habits, time triggers and behavior patterns: These are among the most common triggers for what is perceived as hunger. Overweight people use their eyes to count calories and not their stomachs. They will simply eat what is put in front of them and accept a very large portion as the appropriate amount to eat.

If it's there, I eat it! It may sound crazy that someone who just had a big meal and feels full would pick up a piece of candy or look for a bag of chips in the cupboard. That is why you need to clean out bad foods and snacks from the house. If you don't have it at home, you can't eat it.

5. Thinking about, smelling and seeing certain foods commonly triggers memories of pleasures associated with eating these foods. Viewing appealing foods on television can create hunger pangs, especially when you are tired.

Questions to Ask Yourself If You are Hungry

We know that thoughtlessly grabbing a handful of nuts or a piece of cheese (both high calorie and without portion control), can add two hundred or more calories to your total calorie intake that day. Figure 3.3 shows you six simple questions to ask yourself when you are confronted with hunger.

Figure 3.3 *Questions to Help You Decide if You Are Really Hungry*

Six Questions to Ask Yourself if You Are Hungry

1. Am I thirsty rather than hungry?
2. Did I skip a meal or eat a meal that was too small?
3. Did I eat food/drink with more than 10 grams of sugar?
4. Am I hungry because it's normal to be hungry?
5. Am I hungry because of anxiety, boredom, depression or habit?
6. Is this really hunger at all?

CHAPTER 4

How Foods Can Cause Fullness or Hunger

Low-carb diets are the most successful for weight loss because they depend on protein, which is the most filling, satisfying, and protective against hunger of all foods and drinks. However, not all proteins are equal. Many contain high fats and therefore, high calories. Since most proteins taste good, people often have serious portion control problems with them. Knowing how to sort "good" from "bad" proteins is crucial for your weight loss success even before you contemplate taking any medication.

In this chapter, I will introduce you to the *Rules of Ten for choosing foods that make you full- proteins and avoiding those that produce hunger-carbs.* "Protein is more satiating than fat and fat is more satiating than carbohydrates… Furthermore, there is no clear evidence that high protein intake increases risks of kidney stones, osteoporosis, cancer, and cardiovascular disease." – Arne Satrap M.D. (2005)

Using the Food Label to Choose Filling Foods and Avoid Those Causing Hunger

Food labels are the quickest and easiest way to help you make the "right choices." However, these labels usually contain too much information that is irrelevant to the task of losing weight. At the beginning of any weight loss plan, you need to keep things as simple as possible and concentrate on the four most critical issues: *portion size, calories, carbs, and protein.* As you lose weight and become comfortable with scanning labels, you can think about other diet aspects like cholesterol, fats, and minerals.

The Rules of Ten to Control Hunger & Produce Fullness

The Rules of Ten can be applied to any nutritional label to help you choose the best foods and beverages that produce fullness and avoid those causing hunger.

Protein Rule: 10 Grams of Protein per Portion Will Produce Fullness

The rapid weight loss observed in low-carbohydrate diets is due to substituting high carb foods with high protein foods. When the choice is low-fat foods then the weight loss is accentuated. The protein in cheeses, sausages, fish, chicken, beef, and pork produces fullness for hours. Weight loss expert Dr. David Wiggle wrote in 2005: "A diet high in Protein results in a sustained decrease in calorie intake. The anorexic effect of protein may contribute to the weight loss of low-carbohydrate diets."

Good Sources of Protein

- 3 oz serving of fish (17-21 grams of protein, 100 calories)
- 5 oz serving of chicken or 4 oz serving of beef (40 grams of protein)
- High-protein shake or bar (15-20 grams of protein, 110-170 calories)
- One egg (7 grams of protein, 70 calories)

Other low-calorie, protein-rich foods with easy portion control are low-carb, low-fat cottage cheese, low-fat cheese, ham, sliced turkey as well as fish and white meat of chicken. Figure 4.1 shows the Rules of Ten. The total carbs in this example is 46 grams of carbs less 1 gram of fiber equals 45 net carbs. This food will produce hunger because of high net carbs and protein as low as 2 grams.

Figure 4.1 *Rules of Ten for Hunger and Fullness*

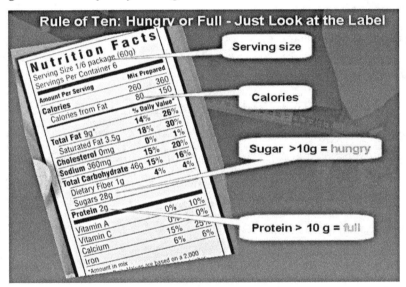

Carb/Sugar Rule: 10 Grams or More of Sugar (or Net Carbs) Will Produce Hunger and Turn to Fat

Ten grams of sugar or more and net carbohydrates over ten grams (total carbs minus fiber carbs) are rapidly absorbed by the stomach, converted to fat, and cause hunger.

Avoid foods and beverages with more than 10 grams of net carbs per portion. Fiber, the parts of plants that our bodies cannot digest, will promote fullness and feelings of satisfaction. (Remember, the suggested fiber intake is 25 grams per day).

"Good" vs. "Bad" Carbohydrates

Selecting foods and beverages that produce fullness is not easy with regards to carbs. The secret is to separate the "good" carbs from the "bad" ones.

Bad carbs: Sugar, fruit juices, candy, cookies, cake, and foods that quickly turn to sugar in the stomach, such as white bread, rice, pasta, bagels, and potatoes.

Good carbs: Most fruits, vegetables and many whole grain bread products, cereals, and even some pasta.

Focus on Fiber-rich Foods

Eating foods with high fiber content can produce feelings of fullness for hours. There are two kinds of fiber, depending on how they dissolve in the stomach. Insoluble fibers do not dissolve and pass through the body undigested. These include wheat and corn bran, whole grains cereals, nuts and seeds, and the skins of some fruits and vegetables. They are frequently used for treating constipation and colon disease.

The other type of fiber dissolves in the stomach, such as the fiber in fruits, vegetables, oat bran, and barley. The more fiber the better. Aim for 25 grams or more of total fiber per day. Vegetables have no restrictions; you can eat as many as you like. Fruits are also a great choice, but bananas, pineapple, and mangos, should be avoided.

Eat a Lot of the "Right" Snacks

Low-carbohydrate, high-protein snacks can avert hunger by preventing sharp spikes and drops in both endorphins and blood sugar levels, which are both hunger triggers. Eating snacks tells our brains that we are not starving ourselves to death. This in turn allows the body to burn more calories. Skipping meals, especially during the day, tells the body to stop burning fat and calories, conserve energy and therefore retain fat stores. The result is failure to lose weight, even in the presence of a reduced calorie diet.

Desirable foods have less than 10 grams of net carbs (the lower the better) and a glycemic index of less than 55. Look for products that are labeled as low-calorie and low-carb, contain non-absorbable fiber, and are sweetened with no-calorie sugar substitutes. The selection of such foods is easier and more attractive every week and includes numerous new soft drinks, some fruit juices, low-carb and low-calorie candy, crackers, ice cream, bread, muffins, bagels, and even pizza.

The Glycemic Index Helps Us Find Foods that Provide Fullness and Avoid Those Causing Hunger

There are numerous naturally occurring good carbs that have little effect on blood sugar, such as fruits, beans, vegetables, and some whole grains. Good carbs are easy to recognize using the Glycemic Index (GI). If after eating a particular food, your increase in blood sugar is equal to what occurs after eating pure sugar, then that carb receives a score of 100 percent. Foods that behave like pure sugar or rapidly turn to sugar have a Glycemic Index of above 55.

Most foods with a Glycemic Index value of less than 55 percent are ideal. These include most fruits, vegetables, beans, whole grain breads, and even some pasta.

Table 4.1 is one of the many Glycemic Index tables available.

Table 4.1 *Glycemic Index of Common Foods*

Glycemic of Common Foods

Low GI	Medium GI	High GI
>55	**56-69**	**<70**
Ginger	Croissant	Brown sugar
Passion fruit	Kiwifruit	Rutabagas
Cucumber	Papaya	Jackfruit
Cherry	Coconut	Nachos
Kidney bean	Muffin	Watermelon
Tomato	Oat	Waffle
Chocolate	Bread	Pomelo
Mixed nuts	Rice	Pretzel
Grapefruit	Pizza	Potato
Pistachio	Common fig	Parsnip
Prune	Persimmon	Beer
Lentil	Wafer	Flour
Eggplant	Honey	Millet
Guava	Breadfruit	Donuts
Lima bean	Melon	Graham cracker
Apricot	Ice cream	Broad bean
Avocado	Raisin	Gingerbread
Strawberry	Beetroot	Mashed potato
Nectarine	Pumpkin	Star anise
Blueberry	Rose hip	Corn syrup
Maize	Pineapple	Amaranth grain

Nutrition Label vs. Front of Product Label

The Front of the Package (FOP) labels describes the product beyond what is required to be listed in the Nutrition Label by the FDA. These are designed to showcase the health benefits of the food and produce a sale of the product. Terms like "low sodium", "high fiber, a "good source of…" "Less sugar" or "few calories" are very common. Many are not regulated by the FDA. Graphics are also used to promote a state of healthiness for the product. All FOP labels are voluntary which leaves space for broad and often unsubstantiated claims.

You can start to apply the Rules of Ten today and for the rest of your life because they are easy to remember, and point you in the direction of the "right foods." In figure 4.2 and figure 4.3, two different yogurts are compared. Yoplait has 14 grams of sugar, 19 carbs and 5 grams of protein and will produce hunger while the Two Good Yogurt with 2 grams of sugar, 3 grams of carbs and 12 grams of protein will make you feel full. With calories about the same, the best choice is the Two Good Yogurt.

Figure 4.2 *High Sugar Yogurt*

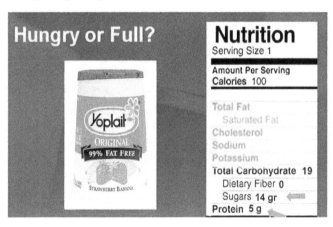

Figure 4.3 *Low Sugar Yogurt*

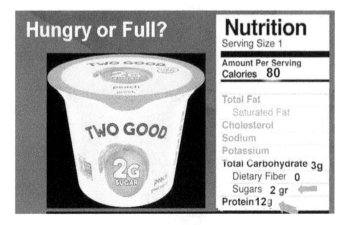

The Rules of Ten for Fullness: Select foods and beverages with more than 10 grams of protein and less than 10 grams of sugar or net carbs, or a Glycemic Index of less than 55 percent to produce fullness and prevent hunger.

CHAPTER 5

How Do Ozempic, Wegovy, Zepbound and Mounjaro Produce Rapid and Safe Weight Loss?

Glucagon-like peptide 1 receptor agonists (GLP-1) belong to a single class of medication but differ in structure, pharmacology, efficacy, and safety. All were initially developed for the treatment of type 2 diabetes. They have been effective not only in reducing blood glucose levels but body weight as well. Mounjaro and Zepbound have a second peptide added to the GLP-1, called GIP.

Indication: As an adjunct to a reduced-calorie diet and increased physical activity for chronic weight management in adult patients with:

1. A body mass index (BMI) of 30 kg/m² or greater. (see chapter 2)
2. A BMI of 27 kg/m² in the presence of one or more comorbidities such as hypertension, type 2 diabetes mellitus, or dyslipidemia.

Liraglutide was the first GLP-1 Approved for Weight Loss

The first of these medications used for weight loss was liraglutide, marketed as Saxenda. Liraglutide has two drawbacks: it delivered only a 5.4% reduction in body weight and had to be administered by injection daily. These drawbacks resulted in the Semaglutides: Ozempic, Wegovy and subsequently Mounjaro and Zepbound.

How GLP-1 Receptor Agonists Produce Significant Weight Loss: Ozempic, Wegovy, Zepbound, Mounjaro

These four medications share a common ingredient: GLP-1, a peptide produced in the L cells of the small intestine in response to food intake which has multiple effects all over the body by their action on GLP-1 receptors. The Tirzepatides Mounjaro and Zepbound have a second peptide, GIP which is made in the small bowel that also controls hunger, cravings, and metabolism. (See figure 5.1)

> **Semaglutides: Ozempic, Wegovy & Mounjaro Control Food Intake by Multiple Mechanisms**
>
> 1. Stimulating Insulin Production
> 2. Diminishing Carbohydrate, Alcohol & Fatty Food Intake
> 3. Slowing Gastric Emptying & Decreasing Food Digestion
> 4. Reducing Appetite and Hunger
> 5. Increasing Metabolism

Tirzepatides: Zepbound and Mounjaro Have a Second Added Peptide: GIP

Tirzepatide, the most recent medication in this class, is more active and potent than the earlier Semaglutides. According to new studies, the GIP peptide, (glucose-dependent insulinotropic polypeptide) produced by the K cells of the small bowel, may be more effective than the original GLP-1 in terms of weight reduction and glucose regulation. In clinical studies, Zepbound and Mounjaro have resulted in weight loss of 25% of baseline weight. This is higher than with Ozempic and Wegovy. They also may have less gastrointestinal adverse effects than the other medications.

Figure 5.1 *Action of Semaglutides in Multiple Organs*

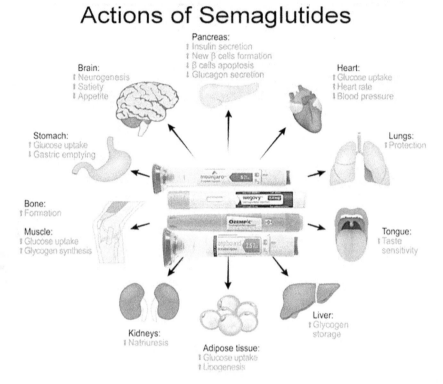

Actions of Semaglutides

Pancreas:
↑ Insulin secretion
↑ New β cells formation
↓ β cells apoptosis
↓ Glucagon secretion

Brain:
↑ Neurogenesis
↑ Satiety
↓ Appetite

Heart:
↑ Glucose uptake
↑ Heart rate
↓ Blood pressure

Stomach:
↑ Glucose uptake
↓ Gastric emptying

Lungs:
↑ Protection

Bone:
↑ Formation

Muscle:
↑ Glucose uptake
↑ Glycogen synthesis

Tongue:
↑ Taste sensitivity

Kidneys:
↑ Natriuresis

Adipose tissue:
↑ Glucose uptake
↑ Lipogenesis

Liver:
↑ Glycogen storage

Actions of GIP Peptide Found in Tirzepatide

When you consume glucose or fat, your body releases many hormones including GIP into your bloodstream. GIP attaches to its receptor on pancreatic beta cells when blood glucose levels are high, causing insulin production. Notably, the impacts on insulin secretion only occur when blood sugar levels are high. GIP does not induce insulin to be produced when blood sugar levels are normal. GIP receptors are also found in fat cells, allowing GIP to promote triglyceride accumulation, and in many areas of the brain. GIP does not have much effect on delaying gastric emptying. Its weight loss effect involves mostly its insulin effect and its effect on GIP receptors in the brain. See Figure 5.2 to see a comparison of GLP-1 and GIP.

Figure 5.2 *Comparison of GIP and GLP-1 Actions*

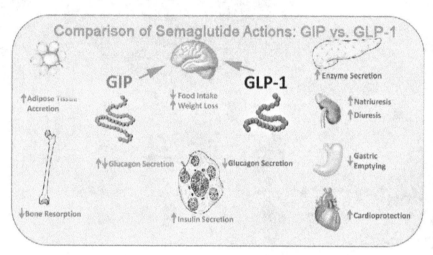

Courtesy: *Baggio,Lauri Glucagon-like Peptide-1 Receptor co-agonists for the treatment of metabolic disease, Molecular Metabolism 46(12):101090, September 2020.*

CHAPTER 6

Weight Loss with Semaglutides: The SUSTAIN AND STEP TRIALS

*T*he *Semaglutide Treatment Effect in People with Obesity (STEP)* program is a group of phase-III studies designed to evaluate the efficacy of once-weekly 2.4 mg Semaglutide given as a subcutaneous injection for treatment of obese and overweight individuals with and without diabetes.

Diet and exercise treatments were incorporated in all STEP trials, albeit at varying intensities. The STEP studies found that high-dose; once-weekly 2.4 mg Semaglutide was effective in reducing body weight in people with obesity and/or diabetes mellitus. Semaglutide had higher gastrointestinal adverse effects than placebo, although it was usually safe and well tolerated. Reduction in carbohydrate and alcohol cravings and preoccupation with eating was noted.

SUSTAIN TRIALS were low doses of Semaglutide (0.5 to 1 mg per week) compared to Exenatide and other diabetic medications in 8000 obese diabetics from 5 countries published between 2017 and 2019. Despite the low treatment doses, Semaglutide-treated individuals lost 3 times the weight as compared to those treated with Exenatide and placebo. In addition, a weight loss response of ≥5% was seen in 52% receiving Semaglutide. Weight loss in SUSTAIN 5 was an average of 13 lb from baseline greater in the Semaglutide 1.0 mg group vs. placebo.

STEP 1 TRIAL was released in The New England Journal of Medicine in 2021 reporting 1961 *non-diabetic* individuals. Semaglutide 2.4 mg per week with lifestyle intervention reduced bodyweight by *14.9%* from baseline after 68 weeks, compared to 2.4% in the placebo group. 86.4% of Semaglutide users lost at least 5% of their bodyweight, and adverse effects included mild to moderate nausea.

STEP 2 TRIAL enrolled 1210 *obese type 2 diabetics* and compared the 1.0 mg Semaglutide dosage to the higher 2.4 mg dose per week and matching placebos over 68 weeks. *Semaglutide (2.4 mg) reduced bodyweight by 9.64%* and placebo 3.42%. Note in this study and many more studies of obese diabetics, weight loss is less in diabetics than non-diabetic obese individuals. This is not unusual because the metabolic abnormalities in diabetics make it much harder to lose weight.

STEP 3 TRIAL had 611 *non-diabetic obese participants with comorbidities* receive Semaglutide 2.4 mg per week or placebo in addition to *intensive behavioral therapy* to support them to adopt a healthier lifestyle. The average weight reduction after 68 weeks of treatment was *16.0%* with Semaglutide versus 5.7% with placebo. The weight loss is similar to that seen in Step 1 individuals.

STEP 4 TRIAL involved *withdrawal of Semaglutide treatment in obese participants with comorbidities.* These 902 individuals all received Semaglutide 2.4 mg per week for the first 20 weeks. At that point, half of the subjects received either Semaglutide or placebo for the remaining 48 weeks. The subjects that had stopped the Semaglutide regained 7% of their lost body weight during the next 48 weeks. Their 68-week weight total loss fell to only 5%. Those that continued with Semaglutide lost 8% more of their body weight, reaching total of *17%* loss. Note how closely the weight loss was at 68 weeks compared to similar studies. *Results showed the effect of withdrawal of* *medication and need for long-term treatment to maintain weight and reach maximal weight loss.*

STEP 5 TRIAL tested the durability of weight loss with Semaglutide 2.4 mg per week versus placebo across a *full 2 years of treatment in 304 nondiabetic obese participants with comorbidities.* Semaglutide resulted in decreasing weight until about week 60 at which time the average weight loss was 15%. The medications were continued thru week 104, during which time the weight loss was maintained at *15.2%.* See figure 6.1 for weight loss results. Note: In the figure, the maintenance of weight loss taking weekly medication extended from week 44 to week 104- a total of 60 weeks.

Figure 6.1 *Two Year (104 weeks) Treatment with Semaglutide 2.4 mg per week (high dose) for Overweight and Obesity in nondiabetics*

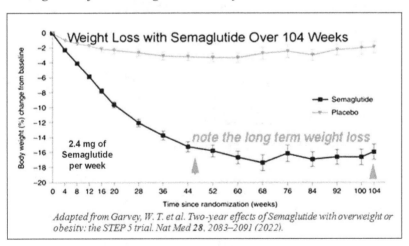

STEP 6 TRAIL focused on Asian people (n=401), specifically those from Japan and South Korea. The researchers found significantly greater bodyweight reductions in people given Semaglutide 2.4 or 1.7 mg per week versus placebo, at *13.2%,* 9.6%, and 2.1%, respectively. Semaglutide treatment also produced a *significant*

reduction in abdominal visceral fat in a subset of people who underwent computed tomography and a significant reduction in AIC in people (~25%) with type 2 diabetes.

STEP 7 TRIAL: not published.

STEP 8 TRIAL compared the weight loss efficacy of Semaglutide 2.4 mg per week against the daily injectable GLP-1 receptor agonist liraglutide at its approved dose for obesity of 3.0 mg. The results showed a significantly greater average bodyweight reduction of *15.8%* with Semaglutide, compared with 6.4% with liraglutide. This equated to average 34 and 15 lb. decreases.

STEP 9 TRIAL using 2.4 mg per week of Semaglutide. The mean change in BMI from baseline to week 68 was –16.1% and 0.6% with placebo. At week 68, a total of 95 of 131 participants in the Semaglutide group had weight loss of 5% or more, as compared with 11 of 62 participants in the placebo group. Reductions in waist circumference, AIC levels, lipids, cholesterol, and alanine aminotransferase were greater with Semaglutide than with placebo.

Summary of Semaglutide Trials

The findings of the STEP trials indicated the efficacy of high-dose, once-weekly administration of 2.4 mg Semaglutide in reducing body weight in individuals with obesity and/or diabetes. Major weight reduction was quite consistent throughout all STEP investigations at doses of 2.4 mg per week despite the distinct characteristics of the behavioral regimens. *The average weight loss over these studies was 14% from baseline.* Semaglutides were shown to have long duration of action, no drug interaction and no negative effects on body functions.

Many of the early trials involved only type 2 diabetics, most of whom were taking medication as well as low doses of Semaglutide

(0.5 mg and 1.0 mg per week). The lower weight loss may be due to the diabetes, the lower dosages, shorter duration of the studies and the presence of other medications (including insulin and others) that may interfere with the weight loss. Despite all of these factors, the obese diabetics were able to lose about 6% of their starting weight with the low dose of 1.0 mg Semaglutide per week. More than 50% lost at least 5% of their starting weight.

These studies demonstrate that, for the first time, there is conclusive evidence that behavioral regimens such as significant exercise and strict food adjustments, which are staples of most current weight reduction programs, *do not* provide any additional advantage to weight loss beyond the effect of the medication. Semaglutide is the medication in this scenario.

CHAPTER 7

Weight Loss with Zepbound and Mounjaro (Tirzepatides), the Dual Peptides: The SURPASS AND SURMOUNT TRIALS

The worldwide burden of obesity and the diseases it causes is rising at an alarming rate. Pharmaceutical methods of weight loss are in the limelight because they go beyond lifestyle changes which have proven after 35 years or more to be ineffective for weight loss and especially for weight maintenance. The goal is not only weight loss but a focus on reducing cardio metabolic problems and prolonging life. (Individuals with BMI of 35 or more have a mortality risk of 2.5 times normal, similar to people with cholesterol of 290 or diastolic blood pressure of 120).

Comparison to Traditional Anti-Obesity Medications (AOMs)

As of 2021, four AOMs have been authorized for long-term administration in the United States: orlistat, phentermine/topiramate, naltrexone/bupropion. Compared to a placebo, the weight loss with currently available anti-obesity medications (AOMs) licensed for long-term prescription usage averages about *3 to 7%*.

Comparison to Semaglutides (Ozempic & Wegovy): Effective Single GLP-1 Agonists Medications

In the previous chapter, a novel injectable medicine, Semaglutide has shown remarkable weight-loss results in a series of global randomized phase III studies. In contrast to the mild to moderate efficacy of current anti-obesity medications (3 to 7%), the average weight loss at maximum Semaglutide dose of 2.4 mg per week was 14%, with one third of persons having a weight reduction of 20% or more.

The primary mechanism of weight loss by Semaglutide is thought to be reduced energy consumption (food and beverage intake) via interference with food preference (especially for cravings and alcohol), inhibition of appetite, and intensification of satiety. Semaglutide also influences energy expenditure and gastric emptying.

Wegovy and Ozempic are the same drug, but with different names and different doses for different conditions. Wegovy is the name of the drug as it's prescribed for weight loss. Ozempic is the name of the drug as it's used for diabetes. The generic name for Wegovy and Ozempic is Semaglutide. Zepbound and Mounjaro are Tirzepatides which contain the same GLP-1 as the semaglutides as well as a second active peptide, GIP. Zepbound is approved for weight loss and Mounjaro for diabetes. Both are still Semaglutides but are included in a subgroup termed Tirzepatides.

Other Differences in the Semaglutides

First, the drugs are made by different drug companies. Competition between these pharmaceutical companies and others that are working on new weight loss drugs may drive down prices for the expensive medications.

Eli Lilly makes Zepbound and Mounjaro while Novo Nordisk makes Wegovy and Ozempic.

Eli Lilly is based in the United States while Novo Nordisk is based in Denmark.

Zepbound, Mounjaro, Wegovy and Ozempic work in similar ways to reduce appetite. But Zepbound and Mounjaro are what's called "dual-agonist" drugs while Wegovy and Ozempic are what's known as "single-agonist" drugs. These drugs activate important hormone pathways in the body.

Tirzepatide is in a completely new drug class. It's a combination peptides. This dual agonist approach seems to cause people who use Zepbound or Mounjaro injections to lose even more weight than those who use a medication that only activates one hormone pathway.

These drugs stimulate hormones that help control blood sugar levels and reduce appetite, triggering weight lossThe hormones are glucagon-like peptide-1 (GLP-1) and glucose-dependent insulinotropic polypeptide (GIP). Wegovy and Ozempic activate the GLP-1 pathway, while Zepbound and Mounjaro activate two: both GLP-1 and GIP.

Zepbound and Mounjaro (Tirzepatide): Dual GLP-1 and GIP Agonists

Tirzepatide is a novel, once-weekly injectable dual glucose-dependent insulinotropic polypeptide (GIP) and glucagon-like peptide-1 (GLP-1) receptor agonist that integrates the actions of the GIP and GLP-1 incretins into a single molecule, representing a new class of medicines for the treatment of type 2 diabetes and obesity.

SURPASS TRIALS: These clinical studies evaluated efficacy of Mounjaro in *diabetics* with and without concurrent diabetic medications. Mounjaro-treated participants had dose dependent reductions in A1C's and body weight and less hypoglycemia than traditionally treated individuals. Weight loss at 5 mg per week was -15%, 10 mg per week dose of -19% *and 15 mg per week dose of -22%.* Average placebo-treated participants lost 3% of their starting weight.

SURMOUNT TRIALS: Surmount-1 studies evaluated obese *nondiabetics* (average weight of 231 lbs.) over 72 weeks with doses of Mounjaro of 5, 10 or 15 mg per week. This group lost 15, 19.5 and 20.9% of their body weight compared to 3.1% for placebo-treated participants. This efficacy is within the range seen with bariatric surgery.

Tirzepatide Weight Loss Related to Dosage:

1. **At the lowest dose**—5 mg per week—participants lost 16 %of their body weight.

2. **At higher doses**—10 and 15 mg per week—participants lost 20% to 23% of their body weight. More than half of the participants taking the higher dose lost 20% of their body weight compared to only 1.3% taking a placebo. *Average weight loss was 52 lbs!*

Trial included type 2 diabetics treated with the weekly 10 and 15 mg Mounjaro (Tirzepatide) doses. All three doses showed significant AIC reductions, and the robust glycemic effect was consistently maintained from week 12 to week 40. Weight reduction in the highest dose was an average of 18 lb. Contrary to the dose dependent reduction in AIC, *no* difference in weight was noted between the 10 and 15mg dose groups. If Zepbound was used instead of Mounjaro the results would have been identical, since they are the same medication.

Zepbound: Tirzepatide Newly FDA Approved for Weight Loss

Zepbound received FDA approval on November 8, 2023, for chronic weight management in adults with obesity (with a BMI of 30 kg/m2 or greater) or adults who are overweight (with a BMI of 27 kg/m2 or greater) and also have weight-related medical problems such as hypertension, dyslipidemia, type 2 diabetes mellitus, obstructive sleep apnea or cardiovascular disease. Zepbound should be used together with diet and increased physical activity.

Zepbound's effectiveness for chronic weight management (weight reduction and maintenance) in combination with a reduced-calorie diet and increased physical activity was established in two randomized, double-blind, placebo-controlled trials of adults with obesity or overweight with at least one weight-related condition.

These studies measured weight reduction after 72 weeks in a total of 2,519 patients who received either 5 mg, 10 mg or 15 mg of Zepbound once weekly and a total of 958 patients who received once-weekly placebo injections. In both trials, after 72 weeks of treatment, patients who received Zepbound at all three dose levels experienced a statistically significant reduction in body weight compared to those who received placebo, and greater proportions of patients who received Zepbound achieved at least 5% weight reduction compared to placebo.

Weight Reduction with Low and High Doses of Zepbound

Patients on Zepbound (tirzepatide) 5mg weekly lost **35.5 lb** on average after 72 weeks. For Zepbound 10mg weekly dose, the average weight loss was **48.9 lb**, and for Zepbound 15mg weekly dose average weight loss was **52.0 lb** over 72 weeks. Patients who used a placebo lost 2.4 kg (5.3 lb) over the 72 weeks. One third of patients lost more than 58 lbs or 25% of their starting weight.

Weight Loss: Ozempic vs. Wegovy vs. Mounjaro

Figure 7.1 compares weight loss between the three Mounjaro doses, Ozempic 1 mg per week, and maximal doses of Wegovy. The Ozempic dose was suboptimal at 1.0 mg. The weight loss might have been greater for the Ozempic group had the maximal dose of 2.0 mg been used in the study.

The disparities in the individuals' baseline characteristics must also be investigated. Patients in SURPASS-1 had a shorter duration of type 2 diabetes, a lower average body weight, a lower mean A1C level, and a lower fasting plasma glucose level than those in STEP-2 or SURPASS-2 trials. Furthermore, the diabetes medications utilized before the study were different.

The Tirzepatides are more effective but results are limited by population differences. Nonetheless, comparisons of Semaglutide and Mounjaro (Tirzepatide) in comparable circumstances are unavoidable and the evidence suggests that Mounjaro (Tirzepatide) is a more effective drug at maximum and even minimum approved doses in both glucose control and weight loss as compared to Wegovy and Ozempic. This most likely is due to the added GIP molecule to the Tirzepatides. Similarly, Zepbound, with 2 hormones, is more effective for weight loss than the single hormone based Wegovy.

Figure 7.1 *Comparisons of Weight Loss Between Mounjaro, Wegovy and Ozempic (adapted table)*

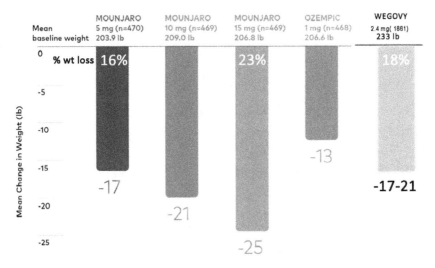

Semaglutide: Comparisons of Weight Loss

CHAPTER 8

How to Use Semaglutides For Maximal Weight Loss

Semaglutides including Ozempic and Wegovy whether used for diabetes or weight loss are a chain of 41 amino acids, as seen in figure 8.1. Semaglutide is a glucagon like peptide 1 (GLP-1) receptor agonist. The Tirzepatides both Mounjaro and Zepbound are peptide molecules that are produced synthetically that acts on both GIP and GLP-1 receptors as receptor agonists. Due to this unique dual activity property, they are also referred to as 'twincretins'.

What are Semaglutides and How Are They Injected?

These medications are injected in small amounts by the individual once a week with an automatic pen injector under the skin usually on the same day of the week. This is called a subcutaneous injection. See Figure 8.2. The injection sites are usually the abdomen but can be in other areas as seen in figure 8.3. Many individuals will rotate injections every other week between the right and left of the belly button. There is no evidence of increased effectiveness by injecting in one area or another. After injection, the Semaglutides are quickly absorbed into the circulation and spread throughout the body attaching to receptors in the brain, stomach, liver, heart, and pancreas.

These medications exert their effect by activation of these receptors. Activation results in the release of chemicals that have multiple effects including decreasing appetite, stopping cravings, and producing feelings of fullness and lowering blood sugar when elevated as in diabetes.

The naturally occurring human GLP-1 is a chain of amino acids called peptides. Synthetic GLP-1 as in Ozempic, Wegovy, Zepbound and Mounjaro are produced by substituting different amino acids at different locations on the chain to produce other effects. Insulin is an example of a well-known peptide. Most people are aware that it cannot be taken orally since it is rapidly inactivated by stomach acids and enzymes thus requiring injections. Peptides have more powerful effects than oral or topical drugs because they are swiftly absorbed by the body and delivered directly into the circulation where they can quickly reach all the organs. The Semaglutide molecule is seen in figure 8.1. The drawing shows Semaglutide is 94% similar to the natural peptide with substitutions where indicated.

Figure 8.1 *Semaglutide Molecule with 31 Amino Acids*

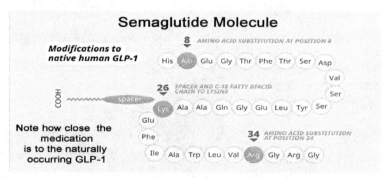

When injecting, the skin and subcutaneous layers are carefully pinched to create a space for the Semaglutide in the subcutaneous layer. However, pinching too hard will have the effect of pushing part of the newly injected liquid out of the body through the needle tract.

Figure 8.2 *Subcutaneous Injection*

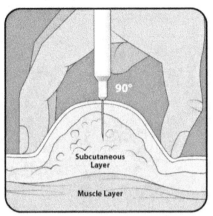

Figure 8.3 *Multiple Areas for Injection of Semaglutides*

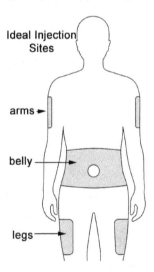

Ozempic, Wegovy, Zepbound and Mounjaro are injected with self-injecting pens as seen in Figure 8.4. When taken weekly by nondiabetic obese individuals, they produce long-term weight loss without significant side effects. In obese diabetics, rapid glucose control is also obtained. Studies suggest greater weight reduction with perhaps fewer side effects with the Tirzepatides. My personal experience is that

Mounjaro has better control of cravings for sweet and salty foods as well as alcohol as compared to the earlier medications.

Figure 8.4 *Self-Injecting Pen*

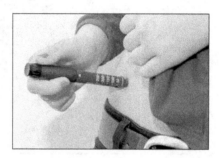

Semaglutide injection with self-injecting pen as with Wegovy and Mounjaro. Each pen delivers a single, predetermined dose and then is discarded.

Long Successful Experience with Ozempic May Predict Results from Wegovy and Mounjaro

1. Semaglutides have Maintained Effectiveness for Years in Individuals with Diabetes

Ozempic has been taken weekly for many years in people with diabetes without losing its effectiveness. Dosing does *not* have to be increased due to loss of effectiveness of the medications as occurs with many weight loss medications. In addition glucose control and the reduction in carb cravings and disinterest in alcohol does *not* appear to diminish over time.

2. Semaglutides are Well-Tolerated over the Long-Term with Few Significant Side Effects

The most common side effects are nausea and mild gastrointestinal symptoms, and these tend to lessen and/or disappear over time. Most patients become acclimated to Semaglutides over time and thereafter have little or no side effects. Any remaining nausea in most patients simply is seen as an annoying nuisance. Re-adjusting maintenance dosing can decrease side effects in those few patients that still have any of the few side effects remaining. For example, Ozempic could be split into two doses taken twice a week.

How Semaglutides are Supplied

Semaglutides including Ozempic, Wegovy, Zepbound and Mounjaro are supplied in pen injectors. Ozempic, being somewhat older uses a pen with an adjustable dose dialer so a single pen can last for 4 to 8 weeks depending on the dose. Wegovy, Zepbound and Mounjaro are sold in single, fixed doses (See figure 8.5). Each pen is used once and discarded. They are purchased in boxes of four pens each with the same dose. Each box is enough for a month. Injections are once a week on the same day of the week.

Figure 8.5 *Semaglutide Injector Pens: Mounjaro, Zepbound, Wegovy &*
Ozempic (Images from sample packages)

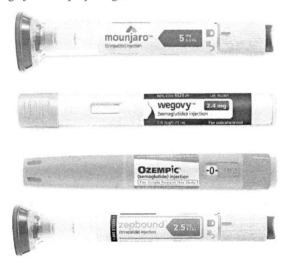

Important Considerations When Starting and Titrating Doses of Semaglutides—Applies to All Preparations

1. **Lowest Dose:** The lowest dose is where to start. For Ozempic/ Wegovy, it's usually 0.25 or 0.5 mg per week; for Zepbound and Mounjaro, its 2.5 or 5.0 mg per week. Sensitive individuals may start at the lower dose.

2. **Dose Titration**: The dose can be raised once a month or even faster with Ozempic, if appetite and cravings are not controlled.

3. **Slow Down in Weight Loss:** The rate of weight loss is dependent on starting weight, age, and gender. Weight loss also slows down normally as weight is lost due to the body's attempt to prevent further weight loss. For example, someone who has had a 30 lb. weight loss would expect to lose at a slower rate than someone who has lost only 5 lb., everything else being equal. There are many other causes of slow weight loss described in Chapter 15.

Therefore, raising dosage simply without evaluating other possibilities for a slow weight loss can lead to more side effects and more problems with cost and availability during the later parts of the weight loss program.

How to Use Ozempic for Weight Loss

Ozempic was released for treatment of diabetes in 2018 as one of the few early once a week injections. After it became apparent that diabetics were losing large amounts of weight, higher doses were evaluated extending the maximum dose from 1.0 mg per week injection to 2.0 mg per week injection. Ozempic is approved for diabetes and is used "off label" for weight loss.

Ozempic is supplied as a single monthly injector pen with a variable dose. Doses are obtained by rotating a dialer on the right end of the pen. Pens are supplied with total doses of 2 mg, 4 mg and newly introduced 8 mg pens. Since the prices for the lower and higher dose pens are similar, I suggest always buying the highest dose pen available. Doses below 1 mg on the 4 and 8 mg pens are not marked but can be achieved by rotating the dialer of the pen on the right and counting clicks.

Using Ozempic with Different Pens Strengths: How to Count "Clicks" for Lower "Microdosing"

a) **2 mg Ozempic pen:** this is the sample pen and is marked in 0.25 and 0.5 mg intervals. It's easy to dial those doses. *Avoid this pen because you can buy a 4 mg or even 8 mg pen at about the same price.*

b) **4 mg Ozempic pen:** this is the most common pen and is marked in 1 mg intervals. Doses below 1 mg are achieved by counting "clicks" as you turn the wheel on the right: 20 "clicks" are 0.25 mg, and 40 "clicks" are 0.5 mg. (There are 19 "clicks" between 0 and 0.25, and 18 "clicks" between 0.25 mg and 0.5 mg) Once you have reached the 1 mg dose, you will see the doses on the dial in 1 mg intervals.

b) **8 mg Ozempic pen:** recently introduced, the pen comes with 2 mg intervals injections marked off on the dialer. Lower doses need to be achieved by counting "clicks". 1 mg is 36 "clicks", 0.5mg is 18 "clicks" and 0.25 mg is 9 "clicks" of the rotating dialer. Figure 8.6 shows the dosing for Ozempic and Wegovy pens.

Figure 8.6 *Titration Schedule for Ozempic and Wegovy Pens*

Ozempic/Wegovy Dosing ↟ dose every 4 weeks				
Weeks 1 2 3 4	5 6 7 8	9 10 11 12	13 14 15 16	**17+**
Weekly Dose 0.25 mg	0.5 mg	1.0 mg	1.7 mg	2.0 2.4

The 17+ doses are 2.0 mg for Ozempic and 2.4 mg for Wegovy.

Adapted from: https://uspl.lilly.com/mounjaro/mounjaro.html#ug0

Starting the Dosage Titration of Ozempic or Wegovy

When using Ozempic, a few dieters start with the 0.25 mg per week dose. After 2 to 4 weeks on the very low 0.25 mg dose, the dieter can progress to the 0.5 mg per week dose depending on side effects and weight loss.

Most people, however, start with the 0.5 mg per week dose for a month or more. Increasing the dose monthly above 0.5 mg depends on the response. Many of my patients do well on the low dose of 0.5 to 1.0 mg per week. There is no reason to raise the dose if weight loss is acceptable and side effects are mild. Remember, most GI side effects occur when increasing the dose. In addition, side effects become milder and milder as the medications are taken.

Need for Higher Dosages of Ozempic in Some Individuals

If you are not experiencing control of hunger on the lower doses, then after a month, it's time to move to the higher doses. Following the titration schedule, you can increase every month until your appetite and cravings are controlled. I believe you do not need to go the highest doses if you are losing weight on the lower doses.

On the other hand, the method outlined in the prescribing guide from the Ozempic and Wegovy manufacturer has the patients increasing the dosage every month until they reach the maximum dose of 2.0 mg per week for Ozempic and 2.4 mg per week for Wegovy.

When using Ozempic, it is possible to split the dose into two injections taking the doses a few days apart. This can potentially reduce side effects.

How to Use Semaglutide Wegovy for Weight Loss

When it became apparent a few years ago that Ozempic could not only treat diabetes successfully but also had a significant weight loss effect, especially at doses beyond 1 mg per week, the Semaglutide in Ozempic was packaged into higher doses in a self-injecting pen and re-named Wegovy. This was approved by the FDA for weight loss. *Note: Ozempic and Wegovy are the exact same medication, with the same dose and scheduling except for the addition of a higher 2.4 mg dose in Wegovy.* Wegovy is supplied in four self-injecting pens per box. Each pen contains a single injection, is used once and then discarded. Boxes of Wegovy pens are seen in figure 8.7.

The medication is in a small chamber buried inside the pen. There is a window to check for color and clarity. A tiny 32-gauge needle for Wegovy and Mounjaro is embedded in the pen, springs out, injects the medication, and retracts. You never see the needle or injection process.

The only difference between Wegovy and Ozempic is the use of the self-injector pen. Using Ozempic, you can dial in any dose and start with any dose you choose. You can change doses from week to week. While with Wegovy, you are supplied with a box of four pens for a month, all with the same dose. You can start with a box of four 0.25 mg pens or slightly higher with the 0.5 mg pens. I suggest starting with the higher 0.5 mg dose. At the end of the month, you can move to the next higher dose or leave the dose unchanged, depending on the dosing protocol. Similar to the Ozempic, you can advance dose by dose each month or elect to stay on a dose that is working for you.

Figure 8.7 *Wegovy Monthly Injector Pens*

(Images from sample packages)

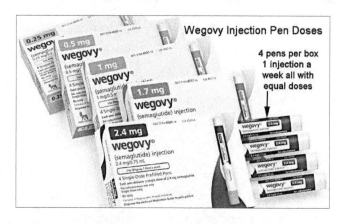

How to Use the Tirzepatides Zepbound and Mounjaro for Weight Loss

Zepbound and Mounjaro, probably the most potent Semaglutide currently available, contain two active peptides—GLP-1 and GIP—that account for its greater efficacy.

They are supplied in a box of four self-injectable pens, enough for a month. Each pen is used for a single injection once a week on the same day of the week.

Like the Wegovy pen injector, the dose is fixed and can only be used once. Doses start at 2.5 mg per pen and increase in 2.5 mg increments to a maximum of 15 mg/pen injection per week as seen in figure 8.8. Weight loss usually starts when taking the 5 mg pen for several weeks. Maximum dosing is the 15 mg pen injected once a week on the same day of the week.

Figure 8.8 *Titration Schedule for Mounjaro Injection Pens*

Zepbound & Mounjaro Dosing ↑ dose every 4 weeks

Weeks	1 2 3 4	5 6 7 8	9 10 11 12	13 14 15 16	17+
Weekly Dose	2.5 *or* 5 mg	7.5 mg	10 mg	12.5 mg	15 mg

https://uspl.lilly.com/mounjaro/mounjaro.html#ug0

I suggest starting at either the 2.5 mg per week or 5 mg per week dosage. Unlike Ozempic but similar to Wegovy, the dose cannot be increased until after 30 days. My experience is that most people do well starting at the 5 mg dose. Doses can be increased monthly depending on weight loss and side effects. Some of my patients can reach their weight loss goals with either the 5 mg or 7.5 mg dosage per week while others require higher doses.

The prescribing guide from the manufacturer suggests increasing the dose every month until the 15 mg dose is reached. My experience both with Ozempic/Wegovy and Mounjaro(and therefore Zepbound) is that similar weight loss can be achieved with lower doses. Recent studies on Zepbound allowed for dose de- and re-escalation during titration to maximize tolerability and weigh loss.

Semaglutide Tips for Rapid Weight Loss with Minimal Side Effects: Best Day(s) of Week for Injections

a) Most of gastrointestinal side effects of nausea, vomiting and diarrhea can be confined to the weekend if the injections are taken on Friday or Saturday. Any nausea, if it were to occur could help limit excess eating and drinking on the weekend.

b) Limiting injections to Saturday may prevent loss of work time if the injections are frequently accompanied by GI side effects.

c) The injection is more effective in the first few days and most people normally eat and drink more alcohol on the weekends. (Semaglutides have potent effects on cravings and alcohol consumption as will be outlined in later chapters).

Switching From Ozempic to Wegovy, Zepbound or Mounjaro

When switching from Ozempic to Wegovy, the *same* doses are used. Zepbound and Mounjaro, however, are slightly different with the added GIP peptide. Doses range from 2.5 and 0.5 mg to 7.5, 10, 12.5 and 15 mg per week. Switching to Semaglutides is more difficult. I suggest those taking 2.5 or 5 mg of Mounjaro or Zepbound to take 0.5 mg of Semaglutide per week. Individuals taking 7.5 or 10 mg should take 1 to 1.7 mg of Semaglutide per week and those taking 12-15 mg of Mounjaro or Zepbound should take 1.7, 2.0 or 2.4 mg of Semaglutide per week.

Fixed Injection Doses of Wegovy, Mounjaro and Zepbound

The Wegovy and Zepbound/Mounjaro pens are simple to use, but because the individual receives four fixed dose pens, the weekly dose can only be changed once a month. Unwanted side effects can only be addressed by skipping the weekly dose or taking medications. Similarly, ineffective doses cannot be changed within the treatment month.

However, it is possible to increase the length between injections which is mildly effective in reducing side effects. In contrast, Ozempic dosage can be changed easily within the month by dialing higher or lower doses.

Splitting Doses within the Week May Lower Ozempic Side Effects

When using Ozempic, it is possible to split the weekly dose into two injections during the week. This is done to reduce GI side effects such as nausea, gas and reflux. For example, a patient taking a 1.5 mg dose of Ozempic per week who has a lot of nausea from the drug could split the Ozempic and take 1 mg on Saturday morning and inject 0.5 mg on Wednesday morning. This does not work for Mounjaro or Wegovy users because of the fixed dosing of the pens. Many individuals find it more effective for weight loss when doses are split.

Which is the best Semaglutide choice? Frequently, the decision boils down to which medication is accessible and least expensive.

SJ has almost completed the weight loss phase. He and his wife from Boca Raton like to enjoy Saturday night parties at country clubs and Boca area activities. SJ is very sensitive to the Semaglutide injections. Doses as low as 7.5 mg per week had significant effects. Taking the injection on Friday or Saturday morning resulted in loss of interest in alcohol and markedly less hunger by Saturday evening. They were unable to enjoy their weekly wine tastings or have a slightly larger dinner with friends. I suggested that he move the injection to Monday morning so that by the following weekend, some of the Semaglutide effects would be less intense.

CHAPTER 9

Low Dosing of Semaglutides and Tirzepatides Optimizes Weight Loss While Reducing Adverse Effects and Costs

The guidelines for taking Semaglutides(Ozempic and Wegovy) and the Tirzepatides(Zepbound and Mounjaro) from the two manufacturers have focused on slowly titrating to the higher doses of 2.0 to 2.4 mg per week of Semaglutides—Ozempic and Wegovy—and 15 mg per week of the Tirzepatides. The rationale for trying to reach the highest dose may be based on using these medications to treat diabetes where the goal is rapidly normalizing blood sugar. This paradigm may not be the best for treating overweight and obese people without diabetes since side effects, and medication availability are all increased with higher doses and the fact that non-diabetics can lose weight faster and more efficient than diabetics.

Rational for Lower Dose Treatment with Semaglutides

During the past two years, I've started treating patients with lower dosages of these medications because of availability problems and increasing costs. Treating with low doses of Semaglutides can encourage compliance and therefore success, especially for those whose insurance does not cover these medications. Just as important, it permits use of lower doses for weight maintenance.

Insurance coverage is an important consideration when taking these expensive medications for long periods of time. Coverage is much more likely for individuals with diabetes than for overweight and obese people without diabetes.

Significant Weight Loss with Low Doses of these Medications

Significant weight loss in even 2-3 months can be achieved by taking low doses of both the Semaglutides and the Tirzepatides. In my experience, using 1.0 mg per week doses or lower of Semaglutide (Ozempic or Wegovy) allows more than half of my patients to reach their target weight. The same effect was seen with treating overweight patients with Mounjaro, where a similar number of the patients reached their goal weight taking the low dose of 5 or 7.5 mg per week of Mounjaro. This can reduce medication prices by half or even two thirds and reduces availability issues. What has applied for Mounjaro should be seen with Zepbound since they are identical medications.

Successful Low Dose Weight Loss is Supported by Two Important Studies:

A. Weight Loss with Low vs. High Doses of Semaglutide

A recently released study (presented in figure 9.1) from the Mayo Clinic compared weight loss in 98 low doses (0.25, 0.50 and 1.0 mg per week) and 77 high doses (1.7 and 2.4 mg per week) nondiabetics treated with Semaglutide after 3 and 6 months. Unlike the results presented in the studies previously, these were patients treated in a normal medical office environment with individualization of doses. The results seen in Figure 9.1 show those individuals taking the low doses of Semaglutide lost *9.2%* of their weight after 6 months of therapy as compared to *12.1%* in those that took the high doses of Semaglutide. Some of the lower overall results found in the studies may be due to the much shorter duration of treatment (3-6 months vs. 1 to 2 years).

Figure 9.1 *Weight Loss with Low Dose vs. High Dose Semaglutide in Non-Study, Non-Diabetic Obese Individuals at the Mayo Clinic*

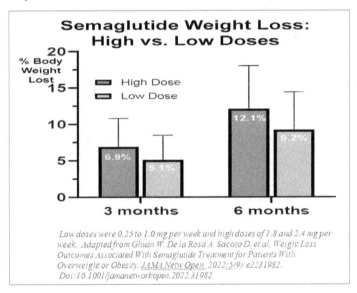

Low doses were 0.25 to 1.0 mg per week and high doses of 1.8 and 2.4 mg per week. Adapted from Ghusn W, De la Rosa A, Sacoto D, et al. Weight Loss Outcomes Associated With Semaglutide Treatment for Patients With Overweight or Obesity. JAMA Netw Open. 2022;5(9):e2231982. Doi:10.1001/jamanetworkopen.2022.31982

B. Weight Loss with Low vs. High Doses of Tirzepatide

In a report in 2022, various doses of Tirzepatide were compared during 72 weeks of treatment. Note that the low dose 5 mg per week group lost 16% (34lb) of their weight by 72 weeks and the high dose 15 mg per week lost 23% (49 lbs). The values apply to both Mounjaro and Zepbound.

Table 9.1 *Weight Loss with Low and High Doses of Mounjaro*

Weight Loss with Mounjaro			
Dose	20wk	36wk	72wk
5mg	11%	14%	16%
10 mg	13%	13%	22%
15mg	13%	18%	23%

Note the very significant weight loss with the lowest Mounjaro dose of 5 mg per week, i.e., a loss of 16% from starting weight at 72 weeks of treatment. Also note the very little difference in weight loss between the 10 mg and 15 mg dose groups. Increasing the dose from 5 mg to 15 mg did have a significant effect on weight loss. More recent data from Surmont 3 published in October 2023 found an average of 49 lb weight loss which was 21% of starting weight. No lower dose groups were included in the most recent studies.

Figure 9.2 *Weight Loss with Low and High Dose Mounjaro (5 mg to 15 mg per week)*

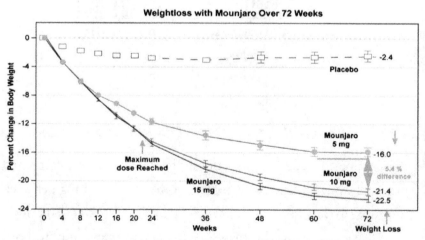

Adapted from Ania M. Jastreboff, M.D. et al. https://www.nejm.org/doi/full/10.1056/NEJMoa2206038

The Case for Trying Low Doses

Many patients (and some doctors) mistakenly assume that taking a higher dose of Semaglutides will lead to much quicker weight loss. Although this is often the case, it ignores the significant number of individuals who can lose a great deal of weight with doses of 5 mg per week of Mounjaro', Tirzepatide and 0.5 mg or 1 mg per week of the other Semaglutides. Note in Figure 9.2 the difference in weight loss of 16% with 5 mg dose and 23% with 15 mg dose after 72 weeks of treatment. There is potentially a great difference in side effects between the two doses. Note that at 60 weeks of treatment in figure 9.2 again a flattening out of the weight loss.

The data presented clearly show that successful weight loss can be obtained taking "low" doses of the Semagltuides and Tirzepatides.

Successful weight reduction with modest dosages of these medications not only minimizes side effects and costs but also encourages overweight and obese people without insurance to seek new pharmacologic therapies that were previously rejected due to poor results of previous weight loss medications or were too expensive or difficult to obtain.

CHAPTER 10

Semaglutide Weight Loss Benefits

Most individuals know the importance of achieving and main-taining a healthy weight. However, not everyone is aware of the unique health benefits of losing weight. Why is it critical to under-stand the advantages of maintaining a healthy weight? For one thing, if you're overweight or obese, that information may motivate you to begin a weight loss program. After you've started a program, remembering the benefits of reducing weight might help you stick to the plan.

Motivations to Lose Weight: Eliminating or Improving Comorbidities of Obesity

It is not simple to lose weight. However, the more you concen-trate on the health benefits, the simpler it is to reach your weight loss targets. There are several reasons to achieve and maintain a healthy weight. Some of the most significant reasons is that weight loss decreases the work of the heart, lowers blood pressure, prevents, improves and often eliminates diabetes, lowers stroke risk, increases mobility, and improves arthritis and cancer risks. Due to a reduc-tion in sleep apnea, fatigue and energy are improved. Not all of the advantages of losing weight are physical. Changes in your self-esteem are likewise significant and should be recognized and appreciated.

How Much Weight Loss is Needed to Improve Comorbidities of Obesity?

Up until a few years ago, before the arrival of new medications such as the Semaglutides, a generally accepted goal of a weight loss program was a 5% weight loss from baseline. The US Food and Drug Administration adopted the "5% or greater weight loss" as the goal of weight loss medications.

The 5% weight loss became the accepted standard of comparison of weight loss results and often the goal of most programs. This was based on statistics from studies in 1999-2001 where a 5% weight was shown to lower BMI and reduce mortality. Widespread adoption of the 5% goal may have been also due to the fact there have been few medications able to produce consistently more than a 5% weight loss from baseline in the past, and none of them have been able to help maintain the weight loss beyond a few months. Only bariatric surgery was able to achieve consistently greater results.

Improvement and Elimination of Metabolic and Mechanical Comorbidities of Weight Gain

Since the Semagludies became available, with typical weight loss outcomes ranging from 14 to 23%, the aim of most weight reduction programs has increasingly shifted from improvement to elimination of many of the metabolic and mechanical comorbidities of obesity. These include normalization of blood pressure, blood sugar, cholesterol and triglycerides (fat in the blood) *without* medications as well as improvements in fatty liver and polycystic ovary dysfunction.

Just as exciting are the improvements in the *mechanical comorbidities* related to the actual loss of fat deposits from around the neck, abdomen and legs. This reduction in fat mass results in improvements in sleep apnea, back pain and arthritis of the knees.

A review of the extensive literature reveals that the metabolic benefits require less weight loss and occur sooner than mechanical improvements. Table 10.1 presents some of the health benefits from various amounts of weight loss that can be achieved using the Semaglutides.

Table 10.1 *Health Improvements with Varying Degrees of Weight Loss*

% Weight loss from baseline	Health Improvements Seen with Weight Loss
0-5%	Lowering blood pressure, blood sugar, and triglycerides
5-10%	Prevention of type 2 diabetes, improvement in fatty liver & polycystic ovaries, lowering of cholesterol, and HDL increase
12%	Improvement in fatty liver
10-15%	Improvement of cardiovascular disease, sleep apnea, esophageal reflex, osteoarthritis of knees, back and hip
>15%	Type 2 diabetes goes into remission, reduced heart attacks, strokes and heart failure

Moderate Weight Loss of 5 to 8%

On the lower end of the weight loss spectrum, even 5% weight loss ameliorates cardiovascular risk factors such as hyperglycemia, hypertension, or dyslipidemia. This goal was reached in 70% to 80% of patients treated with 2.4 mg of Semaglutide and 15 mg of Tirzepatide injected weekly.

Benefits of Weight Loss of 10 to 12 %

A more significant weight loss of up to 10% to 12% is associated with improvements in obstructive sleep apnea, polycystic ovarian syndrome, elevated cholesterol, and non-alcoholic steatohepatitis.

Weight Loss in Excess of 12-15%

A 15% loss is associated with type 2 diabetes remission and mortality reduction. Approximately 65% of patients treated with Semaglutide 2.4 mg per week or Tirzepatide 15 mg per week experienced body weight reductions of at least 10% and 15% respectively.

Improvements in Metabolic, Body Composition and Mechanical Parameters with Weight Loss

A. Improvement in Metabolic Parameters Occur First

A loss of only a few pounds results in the first change in metabolic abnormalities seen with weight gain beginning with a fall in blood glucose and triglycerides. Diabetics find better control of their blood sugar and pre-diabetes often return to normal. As weight continues to fall, blood pressure, and HDL cholesterol levels normalize. When weight loss approaches 10%, many patients need to reduce or eliminate medications for hypertension and diabetes (other than Semaglutides).

B. Body Composition Changes with Semaglutide-Induced Weight Loss

All anti-obesity medications aim to achieve a healthy body composition rather than merely losing weight. As seen in Figure 10.1, Semaglutides significantly reduce *total body fat* by 17.8 lbs. and lean body mass by 11 lb. *Visceral fat* (fat inside the abdomen) was also reduced. *Fatty infiltration of the liver* as seen in figure 10.2 was reduced by 24.7%. This was observed after 68 weeks of taking a low dose of 1.0 mg per week of Semaglutide. *These results are consistent with previous studies with 1.0 mg per week of Semaglutide, which showed that weight loss with these agents was due to loss of fat mass rather than lean body mass.*

Figure 10.1 *Body Composition Changes: Reduction in Total Body Fat with Semaglutide*

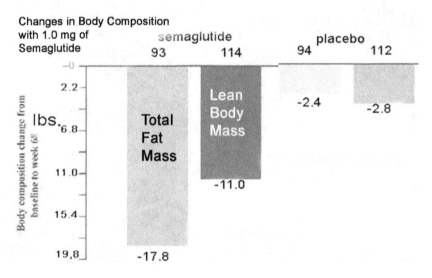

Changes in Body Composition with 1.0 mg of Semaglutide

Adapted: Gastaldelli, Amalia et al https://www.sciencedirect.com/science/article/abs/pii/S2213858722000705

Improvements in body composition may also impact physical functioning. For example, a higher proportion of fat-free mass has been demonstrated to correspond with increased walking ability in obese individuals. The message is that even a low dose of Semaglutide is correlated with improvements in a broad range of metabolic and cardiovascular risk factors, and that even more weight reduction (10-15%) produces even more improvement in these risk factors.

Reduction of Fat Stored in the Abdomen (Visceral Fat) and Liver with Low Doses of Semaglutides

More important than abdominal fat is actual fat infiltration of the liver. In figure 10.2, diffuse fatty infiltration is seen on the yellow-orange areas in the liver MRI on the left. After Semaglutide treatment, clearing of the fat is seen on the blue areas on the right MRI.

Figure 10.2 *Reduction in Fatty Infiltration of Liver with Semaglutides*

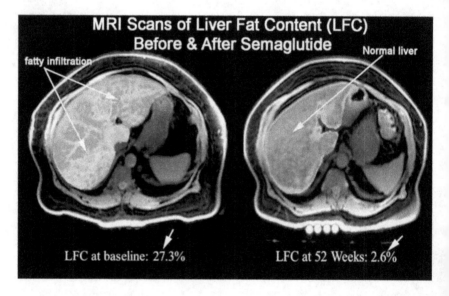

Gastaldelli, Amalia et al. https://www.thelancet.com/journals/landia/article/PIIS2213-8587(22)00070-

Reduction in Fatty Liver in Patients with Non-Alcoholic Steatosis (Fatty Liver) and Non-Alcoholic Steatohepatitis (NASH)

Fatty liver is the most common of the non-alcoholic fatty liver diseases. NASH is just a progressive form with inflammation and fibrosis often leading to cirrhosis and even cancer. It has become the most common cause of chronic liver disease in the developed world.

It has also risen to the top of the indication list for liver transplantation in the United States. Obesity is the cause of fatty infiltration of the liver and eventually NASH.

Two years ago, researchers released a trial of Semaglutide, given *once-daily*, subcutaneously for 72 weeks for the treatment of non-alcoholic steatohepatitis (NASH). The authors found that among 230 NASH patients with fibrosis, 59% of patients with Semaglutide at a dose of 0.4 mg per week had marked improvement compared to 17% in the placebo group. This is the highest response rate that an active drug has ever achieved in treatment of fatty liver and NASH.

Improvements in Mechanical Impairments Due to Reduction in Fat Mass

Reduction in fat mass as a result of losing weight is accompanied by many changes in physical activity levels and mobility limitations. Specific improvement is seen in many body functions including pain, sleep, fatigue and inflammation.

1. Arthritis of the Hips and Knees: In cases of lower extremity osteoarthritis, for instance, every 10 pounds of extra weight causes the stress on the knees during everyday activities to increase by 50 pounds as seen in figure 10.3. Weight loss of even 10-15% can reverse mobility problems, reduce pain by reducing pressure on the spine, hips and knees and prevent progression of the "wear and tear" on these joints.

2. Sleep Apnea Due to Excess Neck Fat: Excess weight creates fat deposits in a person's neck called pharyngeal fat. Pharyngeal fat can block a person's upper airway during sleep when the airway is already relaxed causing sleep apnea. A weight reduction of 7-11% has been noted to reverse sleep apnea.

Figure 10.3 *Obesity and Arthritis of Knees*

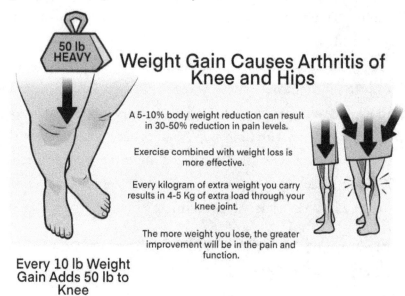

Figure 10.4 *Fat Deposits Reduced with Semaglutide Treatment*

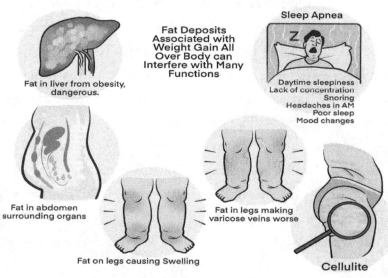

3. Enlarged Fat Masses Release Cytokines (small proteins released by many cells causing inflammation, clotting and often tissue damage): These chemicals circulate all over the body involving distant organs. Fat deposits and their action on various organs is illustrated in figure 10.4. In addition, free fatty acids from abdominal fat deposits are released directly into the portal vein, where they are absorbed by the liver and contribute to abnormal lipid profiles and insulin resistance. All of these metabolic abnormalities are reversed with weight loss.

The message is Semaglutides, even in low doses of 1 mg per week, have potent effects on a broad range of metabolic and cardiovascular risk factors. This includes the common reduction in blood pressure, cholesterol and especially elevated blood sugar in normal people and diabetics. Less recognized is that even more weight reduction (10-15%) produces improvement in complications of the fat depositions in various organs themselves.

CHAPTER 11

Semaglutides Reduce Cravings for Carbohydrates, Fatty Foods and Alcohol

Managing food cravings, especially for sweet and fatty meals encountered in daily life, is critical for weight reduction and long-term weight control. My experience treating patients with Ozempic and Wegovy and later with Mounjaro has shown a significant reduction in cravings for carbohydrates, fatty meals, and alcohol.

This reduction in cravings can be marked and often occurs within a week or two of starting these medications. I have talked with hundreds of patients who tell me their intense desire for carbs in the evening actually disappeared a few days after starting the 5 mg injection of Mounjaro. Gradually they realize they no longer look forward to pasta or rice and seek protein, especially chicken and beef. Often this occurs with low doses and often before they see large amounts of weight loss.

Reduction in Caloric Count of Meals with Semaglutide

Table 11.1 from the STEP TRIAL shows the differences in food intake for each meal with oral Semaglutide treatment. The results are from studies completed in the UK with inpatient individuals in a metabolic ward where food could be measured daily. Note the reduction of food intake varied from 36% to 42% with Semaglutide treatment.

Table 11.1 *Reduction in Meal Sizes with Semaglutides*

Energy intake, kJ	Oral semaglutide	Placebo	
Lunch meal	2133	3331	−35.9%
Evening meal	2620	4546	−42.4%
Snack box	3237	5210	−37.9%
Total daily intake	7991	13087	−38.9%

Adapted from Gibbons et al, Diabetes Obis Metal. 2021 Feb;23(2):581-58. https://www.hejm.org/doi/full/10.1056/nejmoal105816

Changes in the type of foods eaten by individuals taking Semaglutide were also recorded in the inpatient studies and are seen in Table 11.2. Note the greatest reduction is found in the "high fat"

Table 11.2 *Changes in Types of Snacks in Subjects Taking Semaglutides*

Energy intake, kJ	Oral semaglutide	Placebo	Relative difference
High fat and sweet	1431	2337	−38.8%
High fat and non-sweet	578	1054	−45.2%
Low fat and sweet	900	1302	−30.9%
Low fat and non-sweet	329	518	−36.5%
High fat	2009	3390	−40.8%
Low fat	1229	1820	−32.5%
Sweet	2331	3639	−35.9%
Non-sweet	907	1572	−42.3%

Adapted from Gibbons et al, Diabetes Obis Metal. 2021 Feb;23(2):581-588.

and "sweet" groups with 45% reduction in caloric intake of these foods. The snack box in the table above refers to an evening snack box consisting of snacks including sweet, salty and fatty snacks.

Reduction in Meal Size and Cravings with Semaglutides

Control of Eating Questionnaires (measuring control of cravings for sweet and fatty foods, overall hunger, and fullness) were used in additional reports. Food cravings can be influenced by emotion; environmental variables, physical activity, food cues/exposure, and uncontrolled eating habits such as binge eating. The reduced food intake observed with Semaglutide did not result in an increased desire to eat, but instead was associated with improved eating control and satiety.

All the subjects in the above studies noted marked increase in their control of eating and often total disinterest in sweet and fatty foods. In the studies, the appetite and craving reductions were *sustained for 2 years while taking Semaglutides.*

How Semaglutides Reduce Appetite and Cravings

Semaglutides cause weight reduction, in part, by directly activating discrete locations within the hypothalamus and brain stem crucial for food regulation including the reward system and emotional regulation areas of the brain. This might explain why Semaglutide therapy results in decreased hunger and food cravings, as well as improved eating control. The specific action on both homeostatic and pleasure generating mechanisms of appetite regulation, rather than a reaction triggered by nausea or food aversion is the cause of the lower energy intake (food and beverages) and subsequent weight loss. Recent studies show the GLP-1 plays a major role in stress-related eating as well. Areas of the brain affected by Semaglutides are seen in the figure 11.1.

Figure 11.1 *Semaglutides Activate Receptors in Several Areas of the Brain*

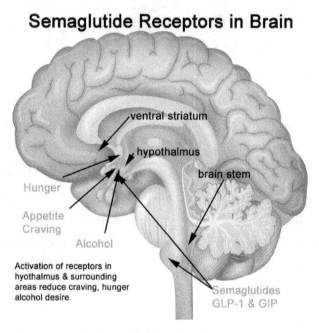

Semaglutides activates neurons in the arcuate nucleus in the hypothalmus called POMC/CART neurons. When activated they reduce food intake and increase energy expenditure. At the same time they inhibit AgRP neurons which when activated increase food intake and decrease energy *expenditure.*

Semaglutides Reduce Alcohol Consumption

Semaglutides reduce alcohol consumption in several ways not only by causing early satiety but by decreasing alcohol's impact on the brain's dopamine production, according to Swedish researchers.

In animal models, Semaglutides including Mounjaro reduce alcohol craving, intake, and relapse drinking. Moreover, studies have shown that the GLP-1 peptide impacts alcohol-related neurochemical reactions indicating that alcohol reduction may result in a decrease in alcohol's rewarding properties.

Mette Kruse Klausen and colleagues reviewed the research on this recently and wrote in the *British Journal of Pharmacology:*

"Studies in rodents and non-human primates have demonstrated a reduction in intake of alcohol and drugs of abuse, and clinical trials have been initiated to investigate whether the preclinical findings can be translated to patients. We suggest that effects of GLP-1 in alcohol and substance use disorders are mediated centrally, at least partly through dopamine signaling, but precise mechanisms are still to be uncovered."

Obese Alcoholics Lose Weight and Markedly Reduce Alcohol

In September 2022, researchers in Denmark released the first study on the impact of Semaglutides in obese alcoholics. It demonstrated lower heavy drinking days and diminished overall alcohol intake in an obese subgroup treated with the Semaglutide, Exenatide. MRIs of the brain of the patients revealed decreased alcohol cue response in the ventral striatum. This is a brain area with a large number of Semaglutide receptors that play an important role in addiction and reward. *This conclusion is significant because it suggests that Semaglutide-treated overweight alcohol drinkers lose cues to reward themselves with alcohol.*

Many patients who have struggled with their alcohol use following the Covid lockdown have experienced a marked reduction in alcohol consumption after only a few weeks on the Semaglutides. It's comparable to what's seen with Naltrexone and alcohol—a complete lack of interest in alcohol. Many of my patients are amazed when what begins as a full obsession with alcohol abruptly vanishes in a few weeks.

JB, a patient of mine remarked several months ago, "What do I drink now? The beer and whiskey are gone. They are not even in my house... In my wildest dreams, I never thought I could go through the weekend without my Coors." I told him to go to 7-Eleven where there is a huge selection of no sugar drinks in single cans and bottles. Buy one of each, maybe a dozen, and find the one you like the best.... Maybe water would be even better.

CHAPTER 12

Adverse Effects and Safety of Semaglutides

The side effects, adverse events and safety issues of the Semaglutides, have been extensively reported in more than 13 separate global clinical phase 3 studies. This includes data from 12,000 participants in the SUSTAIN program and from over 9,500 subjects in the PIONEER trials. With a range of 26 to 105 weeks of Semaglutide treatment, there has been the equivalent of many years of patient follow-up, allowing for a sufficient analysis of the side effects and safety profile of the medications.

Non-specific gastrointestinal side effects are the most common problems accounting for a placebo-adjusted incidence of 11%. Other less common gastrointestinal issues reviewed include possible increase risk for pancreatitis, and gallbladder stones. Less significant have been reports of fatigue, altered taste, hypersensitivity reactions at injection sites and very rare hypoglycaemic (low blood sugar) reactions. Potentially serious adverse effects such as pancreatic and thyroid cancer were not found in any of the studies.

Other problems, such as adverse effects on the cardiovascular system, acute renal damage, and diabetic retinopathy, were addressed early in the development of these drugs and determined to be absent or negligible. Most recent study of Tirzepatides (Mounjaro and Zepbound) found 0.3% of subjects had some Cardiovascular event which was exactly the same as placebo.

Non-Specific Gastrointestinal Adverse Effects

Gastrointestinal disturbances including nausea, vomiting and diarrhea, constipation, and abdominal pain are the most significant and recurring side effects. They have been observed in all of the Semaglutide studies often at different rates and severity depending on the specific population, dosage of medications and the rate of titration. In general, they have a high incidence and a low severity.

Overall, in Ozempic-Wegovy Trials (STEP 2): 88 % of Sema-glutide 2.4 mg per week participants, 82 % of Semaglutide 1 mg per week participants, and 77 % of placebo participants reported experiencing GI side effects. The high incidence in placebo-treated patients and the fact the 2.4 mg and 1.0 mg dosing had almost a similar incidence of nausea, suggests that most of the side effects are quite common, mild and self-limiting. *A placebo-adjusted incidence of non-specific GI side effects was 11 %* (Subtracting incidence in treated patients from placebo). In several STEP Trials non-specific gastrointestinal adverse effects may reach as high as 25%.

The most recent studes with Tirzepatide showed an incidence of nausea of 39% vs. 14% in placebo.

The Mayo Clinic released an updated report on the frequency and severity of patients taking Semaglutides in 2022 which is presented in Table 12.1. This report noted 8.6% of the patients reported moderate side effects and only 2.9% reported severe side effects. Sixty percent of the side effects were gastrointestinal.

Table 12.1 *Non Specific Adverse Effects of Semaglutide Treatment and Their Severity*

Adverse Effects and Their Severity	
Adverse effect	No. (%) (N = 175)
Any adverse effect	85 (48.6)
Nausea and vomiting	64 (36.6)
Diarrhea	15 (8.6)
Fatigue	11 (6.3)
Constipation	10 (5.7)
Abdominal pain	9 (5.1)
Headache	5 (2.9)
Acid reflux	4 (2.3)
Others	8 (4.8)
Adverse effect severity	
None	90 (51.4)
Mild	65 (37.1)
Moderate	15 (8.6)
Severe	5 (2.9)

Adapted from Ghusn W, De la Rosa A, Sacoto D, et al. Weight Loss Outcomes Associated With Semaglutide Treatment for Patients With Overweight or Obesity. JAMA Netw Open. 2022;5(9):e2231982. Doi:10.1001/jamanetworkopen.2022.31982

Same Weight Loss with or Without Gastrointestinal Side Effects

Most important is that weight loss was comparable in participants with GI side effects vs. those without GI side effects. Researchers reported that GI side effects were *not* significant overall factors influencing weight loss although it may contribute to weight loss in some individuals.

Reduce Side Effects with Low Doses of Semaglutide

Notably, higher dosages of Semaglutides are frequently linked with more frequent gastrointestinal side effects. As a result, a dosage escalation system is recommended, beginning with a low dose 0.25 mg or 0.5 mg per week for Semaglutide (Qsymia and Wegovy) and 2.5 or 5 mg per week for Tirzepatides. When rapid dose escalation was employed, 77% of patients reported gastrointestinal side events.

Gastrointestinal Side Effects as Cause of Medication Termination

Despite the mild severity of the gastrointestinal side effects, gastrointestinal problems are the leading cause of medication termination. In one retrospective analysis of 189 individuals with type 2 diabetes who started subcutaneous Semaglutide, 9.5% quit medication due to gastrointestinal issues, while 5.8% had slowed down on their titration.

Data from clinical studies and my experience reveals that about 6 to 8% of patients quit Semaglutide due to gastrointestinal issues. This may be a little lower in those treated with Mounjaro.

Techniques to Limit Gastrointestinal Side Effects

1. Eat slower with smaller portions.

2. Stop eating before feeling full. Some investigators believe that the nausea occurs when attempting to eat on a full or semi-full stomach.

3. Avoid fatty, greasy foods and high carb foods.

4. Medications to Reduce the GI side effects include: Zofran (Ondansetron), Trans Derm Scop, Promethazine, Phenergan, Prochlorperazine (Compazine), and Dramamine.

5. Pre-injection treatment with Zofran (Ondansetron).

Medical Treatment of the Non-Specific Gastrointestinal Adverse Effects

• *Nausea:*

Nausea is clearly the most common GI side effect. It's often seen in the very beginning and during dose escalation, but for most people; it gets less and less significant as time passes. If it occurs early in the week, it's usually the effect of the drug itself. Nausea halfway through the week is usually as a result of overeating. Since nausea can occur in the fasting state, researchers have concluded some of the origin of the nausea may be the effects of Semaglutide on the brain.

Rx: OTC meds like Gas-X, Pepto-bismol, Imodium and prescription Ondansetron (Zofran) orally or Compazine by injection.

• *GERD-Heartburn-Reflux:*

There is a transient worsening or new onset of gastroesophageal reflux disease (GERD; a known complication of obesity) during treatment for many patients. Medications such as proton-pump inhibitors or H2-blockers can be used on a temporary basis.

Rx: Omeprazole (Prilosec-once or even twice a day), for breakthrough pain H2-blockers such as Pepcid AC, Tagamet, Protonix, Prevacid.

• *Constipation:*

This is one of the most common side effects due to the medication or even more likely the change of food. More than 46% of subjects complained of constipation. Treatment includes the usual treatments of constipation.

Rx: Fiber such as Metamucil capsules 2-3 twice a day with several glasses of water, stool softeners and/or Miralax.

• *Vomiting:*

This less common side effect is usually transitory and occurs more in the initial phase rather than with higher doses. Often, treatment for GERD like symptoms can stop vomiting. If severe, then the anti-emetics can help.

Rx: OTC products: Dramamine, Bonine, Gravol, Pepto-Bismol, Emetrol. Prescriptions include Zofran, Compazine, Phenergan

Other Non-Related Causes

Clinicians should also consider whether any existing or recently initiated concomitant prescription or non-prescription medications could be responsible. For example, metformin can cause GI side effects.

Specific GI Adverse Effects: Low Incidence-Moderate Severity

Gallbladder Disease with Semaglutides

When Semaglutides were compared to other diabetic medications and placebo, the Sustain Trials (2016-2021) found 83 individuals (1.4%) on Semaglutide suffered a gallbladder incident, compared to 39 patients (1.9%) on placebo. These results need to be interpreted with the understanding that all the weight loss patients in these studies were diabetics who have a 32% incidence of gall bladder disease compared to non-diabetics. In the 400 patients I have treated with these drugs, I have encountered 3 patients with gall stones requiring *surgery.*

Tirzepatide treated participants in more recent studies (2022 and 2023) had an incidence of gall bladder disease of 0.8% to 1.7%. (placebo incidence was 1%). The most common occurrence again was cholelithiasis. Interpretation is difficult because obese people who undergo rapid weight loss without medications have a 21% incidence of gall bladder problems.

Cause of the Gall bladder Difficulties

Originally, it was believed that gallbladder events were linked to rapid Semaglutide-induced weight loss. Nevertheless, because gallbladder disease is not a problem with other diabetic drugs causing rapid weight loss, and often occurred long after the weight loss period ended, attention has been focused on changes in gall bladder motility and shift in bile salts from the GLP-1 medications.

Symptoms of Gall Bladder Disease

First, most gallstones do not cause symptoms. However, when gallstones become larger, or when they begin obstructing bile ducts, symptoms or "attacks" begin to occur. Attacks of gallstones usually occur after a fatty meal and at night. The following are the most common symptoms of gallstones:

Symptoms may include: pain in upper right of abdomen, fever, chills, Jaundice, bloating, intolerance of fatty food, belching and gas.

The symptoms of gallstones may resemble other conditions or medical problems, such as heart attack, appendicitis, ulcers, irritable bowel syndrome, hiatus hernia, pancreatitis, or hepatitis. Always consult your health care provider for a diagnosis.

Pancreatitis Adverse Events: Very Rare and NOT Caused by Semaglutides

Patients with diabetes who have a reason for GLP-1 treatment frequently have associated risk factors for pancreatitis (notably obesity, longer diabetes duration and co-medication). However, as indicated in the Table 12.2, pancreatitis and pancreatic cancer are very rare and *not* associated with these medications. The placebo incidence exceeded the active medication in 2/3 studies.

When Semaglutides were first tested, they were exclusively used in diabetic individuals, often ones with severe disease. This skewed the data because this group of people have a naturally higher incidence of pancreatitis than nondiabetic obese people. More recent updates indicate in the Tirzepatide treated groups an incidence of 1% which was the same as placebo.

Table 12.2 *Acute Pancreatitis in Semaglutide-Treated Patients*

Semaglutides and Acute Pancreatitis	(cases)	
	Sustain 6	Pioneer 6	Tirzepatide
Treatment	9	1	5
Placebo	12	3	3

Non-Gastrointestinal Adverse Events: Rare and Mild

1. Cardiovascular Effects of Semaglutides: Only Mild Increase in Heart Beat

All Semaglutides raise heart rate, and these drugs are no exception. In SUSTAIN-6 Trials, a placebo-corrected heart rate rise of 3.2 beats per minute for Semaglutide 1.0 mg was seen. This increase was *not* linked to any negative cardiac events or adverse cardiovascular outcomes. In fact, I have never seen a patient whose blood pressures worsened with these drugs. They almost always improve.

At this stage, it is obvious that the favourable benefits of Semaglutides on cardiovascular risk factors and physiology outweigh the danger, if any, of an increase in heart rate.

2. Low Blood Sugar (Hypoglycaemia) Reactions: Only in Diabetics Taking Other Medications

Since control of blood sugar was the initial reason for the development of Semaglutide medications, it is expected that one might see some blood sugar reduction with Semaglutide treatment in non-diabetics. Although it is possible that blood glucose levels will fall, it's a rare complication that it will be significant.

One-third of the patients I have treated report fatigue especially in the first few days after the injection, usually in the late afternoon and often after skipping lunch or an afternoon snack. This is often due to a lowering of blood sugar to lower levels than most people experience. A typical complaint I hear is that a patient who routinely goes to the gym after work at 6 p.m. or goes grocery shopping feels exhausted and is unable to do so.

In diabetic patients taking other glucose lowering medication, the presence of Semaglutide may lower blood glucose levels even more.

3. Fatigue, Lack of Energy, Headaches and Light-headedness: Mild, Often Due to Skipping Meals

Other side effects include fatigue, cold sweats, headaches, dizziness and light-headedness. There are multiple causes for these side effects. Figure 12.1 illustrates the many causes of fatigue and lack of energy.

4. Acute Kidney Injury: Not a Complication

Initial case reports suggested that Semaglutide treatment could cause acute kidney injury (AKI) in some patients. Mechanistically, this was explained by dehydration caused by nausea, vomiting and diarrhea. However, this was not found in further studies. Acute kidney

Figure 12.1 *Causes of Fatigue in Semaglutide-Treated Patients*

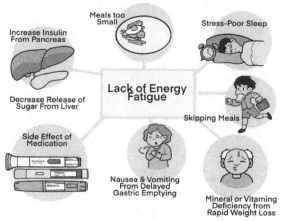

injury was found in 2.0% of patients treated with Semaglutide and 2.3% of placebo-treated patients.

5. Allergic Responses at the Injection Sites

Although any subcutaneous injection can cause injection-site hypersensitivity (allergic reaction), there is no evidence that this is more common with Semaglutides than with placebo. Hypersensitivity(Bruising, redness, induration, and discomfort) at the injection site was observed in 0.6% of the semaglutide groups and 0.8% in the placebo. None of these responses were judged serious. In the more recent Tirzepatide studies from 2023 the incidence was higher at 11% compared to placebo of 1%.

6. "Ozempic Face or Butt:" Wrinkly Skin

These skin changes have been trending on-line, referring to loose or wrinkly skin from rapid or large amounts of fat loss on the face and buttocks. Especially seen in older people it's not really a "side effect" of the medications. Due to changes in skin elasticity, it can often be avoided by slower weight loss.

7. Medullary Thyroid Carcinoma: Only in Rodents

Semaglutides have received an official box warning for medullary thyroid carcinoma. This caution is based completely on information from rodent studies due to high GLP-1 receptor expression in rodent thyroid C-cells.

Three incidents of malignant thyroid neoplasm were discovered in the SUSTAIN program; two in Semaglutide-treated patients (combined n = 5,933) and one in the placebo group (n = 4,736). *They were not medullary carcinomas (MTC).*

MTC is extremely rare (incidence of 2 occurrences per 1,000,000 patient-years), making it extremely difficult to rule out a link between Semaglutides and thyroid cancer. As a result, regulatory authorities mandated extra vigilance. Meanwhile, in the United States, Semaglutide is contraindicated in individuals with a personal or family history of MTC, as well as in patients with type 2 multiple endocrine neoplasia (MEN).

Summary of Adverse Effects of Semaglutides

The Semaglutide family of medications has been associated with a few negative side effects throughout the years, most of which have subsequently been explained in many studies involving thousands of people worldwide. As compared to placebo, Semaglutide causes mostly modest and temporary gastrointestinal symptoms and has a slight increase in the risk of cholelithiasis. There is *no* indication of thyroid malignancy and *no* increase in pancreatitis or pancreatic cancer.

CHAPTER 13

Semaglutide Food Plan for Rapid Weight Loss

The Semaglutide Food Plan is a long-term weight management program that is meant to help you lose weight rapidly with Semaglutide injections and a simple low-carbohydrate, high-protein diet, and then maintain the weight reduction. It is intended to assist you in reshaping your lifestyle by incorporating healthy new habits and breaking harmful old ones. The objective is to make easy, enjoyable modifications that will result in a healthy weight that you can sustain for the rest of your life. Simple dietary changes are offered, such as avoiding missing breakfast, having a protein snack late in the afternoon, and substituting "bad carbs" with "good carbs."

The diet emphasizes three meals each day: breakfast, lunch, and dinner, as well as an afternoon protein snack. This program may be personalized to your specific needs, medical history, and dietary habits.

What is Different about the Food Plan?

A. Unlike other weight loss plans, there are *no* recipes, specific preparations, or grocery shopping. The meal options are displayed in four menus, with thumbnail images of each choice showing portions, preparation, and, in certain cases, calories, carbohydrates, and protein.

B. The Semaglutide Plan is based on the most effective set of weight loss drugs developed to date. Most dieters are not preoccupied with hunger, appetite, or temptations, and often must make a conscious effort to eat and not miss meals. This is especially important late in the afternoon when the lack of hunger and cravings cause many dieters to miss the afternoon meals.

C. Sweet and fatty food cravings as well as alcohol cravings are invariably decreased and often eliminated by the action of the semaglutide medications. This is encountered after only a few weeks of starting the medications, but is often so subtle it's hard to recognize at first.

All the successful dieter needs to do is follow a few easy steps with their food and allow the Semaglutides to assist them.

The Best Dietary Approach to Obtain Maximal Weight Loss and Weight Maintenance

1. Low carbohydrate diet with 50-70 grams of net carbs per day and less than 10 g sugar/carbs per portion encourages fullness and prevents hunger.

2. High protein as possible—usually more than 90 to 150 grams of protein per day and greater than 10 g protein per portion.

3. *NO* intermittent fasting, keto diets or skipping meals.

Here are Some the Factors Making This Diet So Rapid and Successful

1. Loss of Appetite with these Medications

Increased secretion of insulin (which diminishes hunger) and decreased release of glucagon (a potent appetite enhancer) both released by the action of these drugs are one of the determinants of the amount of weight loss.

2. Decrease in Cravings for Sweet, Salty and Fatty Foods

Sugary foods are to be avoided simply because they work against the weight-loss action of the medication. Sugar is calorie-dense and non-nutritious, produces hunger rather than assisting in producing fullness. These include *starchy foods such as white bread, pasta, rice and potatoes, desserts, candy, and sugary beverages including soda, juices and energy drinks.*

3. Delay in Gastric Emptying Time

One of the major effects of these medications is delay in gastric emptying. The stomach remains filled with food for prolonged periods of time causing a prolonged sense of fullness and lack of desire to eat. It is this effect on the stomach that results in some of the weight loss and most of the side effects of these drugs.

4. Activation of Stretch Receptors in the Stomach

Stretch receptors are found throughout the stomach and gastro-intestinal system and respond to GI tract distention by sending signals back to the brain suggesting fullness and the need to reduce food consumption.

Breakfast on the Semaglutide Food Plan

Individuals struggling with their weight are more successful if they have breakfast. It's about metabolism, control and making better choice at lunch. Protein (> 10 grams) is the key to successful control of breakfast and lunch. Best choices are seen in Figure 13.1.

Figure 13.1 *Breakfast Menu on Semaglutide Diet*

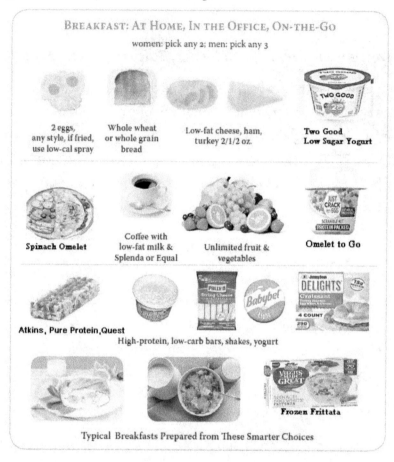

Typical Breakfasts Prepared from These Smarter Choices

Secrets to the Perfect Breakfast: Don't Skip it and Have Protein

1. **Drinking only juice and/or coffee** is the same as skipping breakfast.

2. **Skipping breakfast** leads to poor choices at lunch.

3. **Convenience rules at breakfast**—it's easy to avoid bagels, pastries, donuts, muffins, sugary cereals if there are other easy choices.

4. **Choose foods high in protein and low in carbs:** Protein should be greater than 10 grams and carbs less than 10 grams per portion.

BREAKFAST: Ideal breakfast is 200 calories (women) and 240 calories (men). The breakfast menu shows best choices with calories and carbs. Vegetables and non-tropical fruits are free.

Lunch on the Semaglutide Food Plan

Most people naturally assume weight gain is due to snacking and poor food choices or portion sizes at dinner. Although this may be partly true, the mistakes made at lunch can far outweigh a few bad snacks or a large meal at dinner. Is this hard to believe? Read on. A sandwich, sub, salad, or soup each average about 300-400 calories. Fast foods, fried foods, and hot dishes containing meat, chicken, rice, potatoes, or pasta (a large meal) typically average between 800 and 1,600 calories. The difference is 800 calories or more.

Secrets to a Good Midday Meal: Keep it small and light with *no* rice, potatoes, pasta, beans, or quinoa. Avoid large portions of beef, fish, chicken that look like dinner. Eat foods served cold. Consider the following guidelines:

1. **One Big Meal a Day:** Few people who work inside a building all day can eat two large meals in a single day without gaining weight. So, small lunches—big dinners!

2. **Time of Day:** The time of day when a meal is eaten has no implication on weight gain or loss, so save the big meal for the evening. At least, you have only had a single large meal a day!

3. **Cold Foods:** Foods served "cold" are usually low in calories and have easier portion control—think sandwich or sub, not rice, pasta, potatoes or beans.

4. **Sandwiches and Wraps Make Great Choices.** They have easy portion control, and low calories. High carb side dishes such as rice and potatoes are seldom eaten with salads, sandwiches, or wraps.

Figure 13.2 *Lunch on the Semaglutide Food Plan*

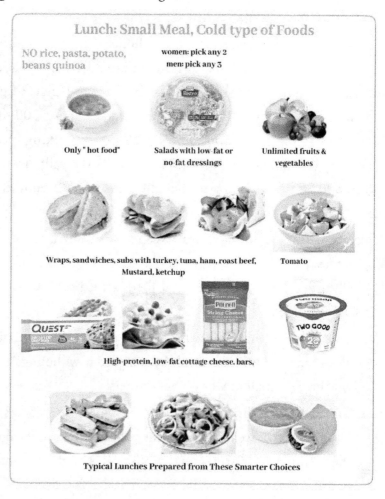

BREADS: *Thin slice, Pepperidge Farm, Nature's Own*

LOW-CARB WRAPS: *Mission, Ole, Joseph, Delicious, Dave's*

SNACKS: *Important, all are low-carb and high protein in portion controlled packages, ideal ones are portable like high protein, low-carb chips (Quest, Puffs) and bars (Atkins, Protein One, Quest)*

Dinner on the Semaglutide Plan: The Large Meal of the Day

Dinner is the large meal of the day. The family sits down together and has this meal. It is an important time to talk about the day's events and future plans. The TV and electronic devices need to be turned off. Even 15-20 minutes set aside for this meal is better than nothing.

The protein and carb part of the dinner is where portion control counts. The biggest challenge to any meal of the day is fast food because of its high-calorie and high carb content. In addition, foods with difficult portion control, such as proteins and carbohydrates, require special attention; the more caloric a food has, the more critical its portion size. Figure 13.3 presents the best dinner choices. Remember, portions are most important when eating beef, pork, and carbs.

Secrets to the Best Dinner: Avoid fast foods, fried foods, and sizable portions of meat and chicken. Have pasta, potato or rice *three* days a week and never, never at lunch.

1. **Dinner should be the big meal** of the day; it's time to relax and eat with family.

2. **Unlimited items:** Many items are completely or almost unlimited, including soups, salads, and vegetables (served without butter or with low-fat or fat-free salad dressings) and most fruits, except for tropical fruits and avocado.

3. **Choose baked, barbequed** or grilled entrees, not breaded dishes. NO FRIED or FAST FOODS.

4. Be careful with proteins and carbs that have portions difficult to control.

Figure 13.3 *Dinner on the Semaglutide Food Plan*

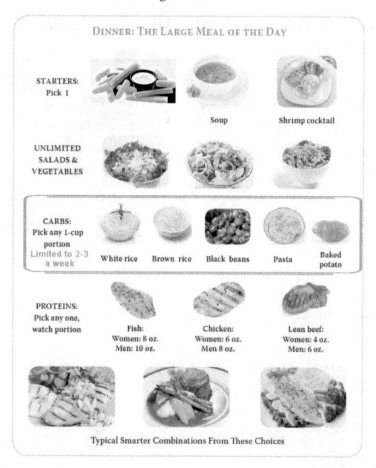

DINNER: The larger meal of the day with unlimited fruits, vegetables, fish, chicken and limited beef and pork. Carbs limited to 3 days a week. Cauliflower rice and potatoes unlimited. Try to eat the protein first and the sides later to prevent fullness early in the meal.

Snacks on the Semaglutide Food Plan

Snacks can save your day, so you need to know the best snacks to prevent hunger and provide satisfaction. The key to the best snacks is portion controlled containers containing less than 10 grams of sugar and carbs and more that 10 grams of protein. The most important snack is late in the afternoon to prevent fatigue and weakness due to low blood sugar reactions as well as to prevent overeating at dinner. The best snacks remain the high protein low sugar bars because of their high protein, portability and satisfaction of cravings. The need for snacks will keep decreasing as well as the cravings due to the effects of Semaglutides on the appetite centers in the brain.

Figure 13.4 *Snacks on the Semaglutide Food Plan*

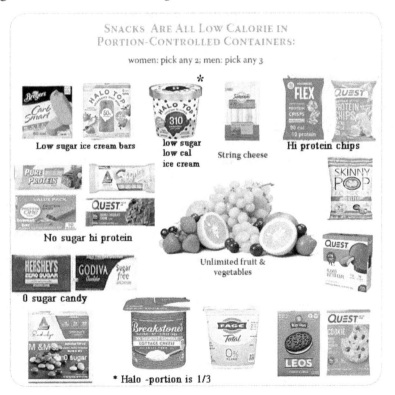

Benefits of Snacking

a. **Binge control**: Snacking on a high-protein bar, yogurt, hard-boiled eggs, or small high-protein zero sugar shakes prevents falls in blood sugar, especially during the late afternoon. Since most fruits are free all day long, eat apples, oranges, and pears which you can find even at a gas station.

b. **Extra energy and nutrients**: Snacking fits our busy lifestyles, offers flexibility, and helps reduce hunger. Healthy, grab-and-go snacks can be a good source of nourishment. Snacks will arm you with an option to prevent hunger and feelings of deprivation if they are the right snacks at the right times of the day. Look for small portion-controlled bags of low-carb chips, crackers, ice cream-like bars, cheese, and yogurt. Seek containers where the portion is 100-130 calories, with sugar and carbs less than 10 grams and protein more than 10 gram per portion. Seek only 1-2 snacks a day.

Minimum Meal on this Plan

It's very easy to start skipping meals on this plan because of the lack of hunger and cravings. Often the dieter ends up with a single large meal a day, usually in the evening. This leads to marked increase in gastrointestinal side effects including nausea, vomiting and abdominal pain often from reflux. Eating three small meals leads to less side effects and greater weight loss. Figure 13.5 shows the "minimal meal" to sustain blood sugar. Note all of the choices contain protein and have few carbs.

Figure 13.5 *Minimal Meal to Sustain Blood Sugar and Prevent Hunger*

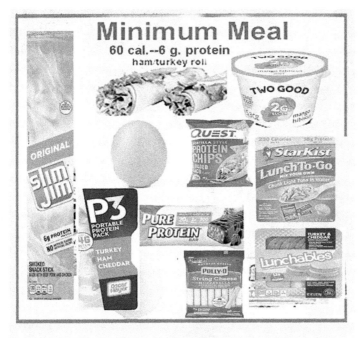

CHAPTER 14

Out of Control Food and Drink Portions

Between 1977 and 2000, portion sizes doubled, and have since tripled for salty snacks, desserts, soft drinks, fruit drinks, French fries, hamburgers, cheeseburgers, and Mexican food. The increase in "acceptable" portions has almost completely mirrored the increase in obesity not only in adults but in children. Figure 14.1 shows how portions have increased over the past twenty years.

Figure 14.1 *Changes in Portion over the Past Twenty Years*

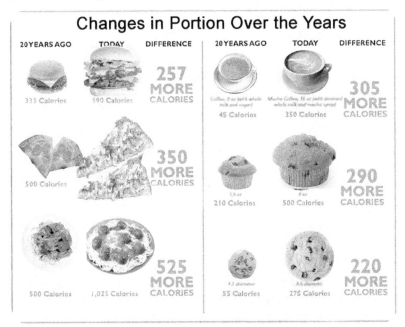

The 8 oz. bottle of soda was the standard size for decades, until it was overtaken by the 12-ounce can. Many stores now carry only 20-ounce soda or juice bottles, which contain 2.5 servings. That one bottle can top out at 250 calories and contain 65 grams of sugar.

Increased Portion = Increased Consumption

A 2004 study published in the journal Appetite gave people potato chips packaged in bags that looked the same, except they were presented in increasing size. As package sizes increased, so did consumption; subjects ate up to 37 percent more with large bags than they ate when presented with smaller bags. Those eating the smaller amount of chips stated that they were just as full as those eating the large amount. Buying groceries in super-sized boxes or bags, or using oversized plates or glasses only makes portions greater. Complicating this is the fact that people seriously underestimate the calories in large portions by as much as 30-50%. Since the amount consumed is proportional to the portion, making these mistakes can cause serious problems.

Portion Distortion Affects Everyone

An obesity seminar for doctors and dietitians was held in Boston a few years ago. After the symposium, self-service ice cream was available. Everything was small in one part of the room—small containers of ice cream, small serving spoons, small eating spoons and small dessert plates. On the other side of the room, the doctors and dietitians were offered ice cream from large containers, using extra-large serving spoons.

Uniformly, the professionals ate 50% more ice cream when using the large as compared to the tiny spoons and containers. No one can get portions right, no matter who you are!

Small Bags and Small Plates Lead to Less Eating

Visual estimates of appropriate portion size can even depend upon how food is served. For example, in a study by Dr. Brian Wansink, diners in two different all-you-can-eat Chinese buffets in two separate cities ate 54% more food when given a 12-inch plate vs. a 10-inch one.

Movie goers were given large and small bags of popcorn. It did not matter which bag each person received—50% asked for more!

Degree of Hunger Does Not Correlate with the Portion

Even more troubling is that it does not matter if a person is hungry or not—they will eat the same amount. Dr. Wansink writes, "If a person generally eats eight oz. of pasta for dinner, they may be quite content eating 6 to 10 oz. of pasta without feeling either overly hungry or full."

Although people could use scales or measuring cups, "people don't like to," says Laurie Acosta, one of the researchers.

"No one is immune to serving size norms—not even intelligent, informed people who have just had a course on the subject," emphasizes Dr. Wansink.

Compensatory Eating is Found Only in Young Children

One might expect that if people eat more during one meal or have a snack, even a substantial one; they will eat less at the next meal. This is called compensation and, it only occurs in 3- or 4-year-old children.

Increased portion size causes increased fullness for no more than 20 or 30 minutes. Over 50% of overweight people are habitual plate cleaners, and the acceptable portion is whatever they see in front of them. Whatever is on the plate is the amount they eat and the amount of food they expect to make them feel full. The intake increases when the food or drinks happen to be pleasing, calorie-rich, salty, fatty, or sweet. Most people—children and teens included—eat with their eyes, not their stomachs.

Portion Size is Not a Popular Subject

With the apparent link between increased portion size and the out-of-control obesity crisis, one might expect that numerous studies have evaluated the long-term benefits of portion control on weight loss and maintenance. However, only a few studies have been done. The emphasis has been on the trendier low-carb or high-protein diet plans, not on the more mundane exploration of portion size.

Portions Can Be Controlled More Easily Than Trying to Limit Foods or Strenuous Exercising

Dr. Everett E. Logue, Ph.D., reported in Obesity Research in 2005 that the most significant study he'd completed was in one that emphasized portion control:

"Although we saw similar patterns of weight loss related to reduced dietary fat consumption, increased fruit and vegetable consumption, increased physical activity, and increased planned exercise, the target behavior that induced the greatest weight loss was portion control."

Dr. Logue adds that exercise was much less critical." Portion control may be *behaviorally easier to change* than increasing planned exercise for many obese individuals." Logue said.

Strategies for Controlling Portions: Semaglutide Reduces Portions

Semaglutide medications make portion control much easier because of the marked decrease in gastric emptying time automatically results in portions that are ½ to 1/3 the size of normal. In addition there are other strategies individuals use to control portions—some are simple, while others are more complex. Incorporate as many as you can into your weight loss plan.

1. Limiting Portions by First Eliminating a Few Exceptionally Bad Foods with Impossible Portion Control

Controlling portion sizes of pleasurable foods using willpower alone is very difficult, especially in times of stress. Intending to eat just a handful of nuts or one scoop of ice cream can result in massive portions. A handful of nuts easily equals 150 calories and many people will eat handful after handful.

Ice cream, cookies, candies, nuts, chips, seeds and cake have NO easy portion control, except when bought in discrete packages such as the 100-calorie packages or for ice cream in 60 to 100 calorie bars.

2. Limiting Portions by Choosing Foods with Easier Portion Control

Some foods have easier portion control than others. When everything is equal, choose the ones with low calories and carbs and easier portion control. A frozen, sugar-free, ice cream bar with 60-80 calories and 3 grams of sugar is a much better choice than a handful of dried fruits, nuts or seeds, because the portion is the entire bar. Getting up for a second and going to the freezer takes more effort than reaching into a bag of nuts, dried fruits, or seeds for another handful. The simple concept is to make the snacks "harder to get".

3. Supermarket Tricks to Aid in Portion Control

The secrets for good portion control start in the supermarket. Buying foods with easy portion control makes limiting food intake much easier when you come home. After you have eliminated the high calorie foods that cause problems, the next step is to control how much you and your kids eat of *other* foods.

4. "Packaged Foods" are not Always "Processed Foods"

I call the foods purchased at a supermarket in bags, boxes, or other containers with nutritional labels "packaged foods." They may or may not be "processed foods." When confronted with packaged foods, the simple trick is to choose the foods where the package itself is the whole portion. Remember that portion control starts at the supermarket, not at the dining table.

Make things easy, so you only need to be concerned with portion sizes for one or two items a day, ideally for protein and carbs you have at dinner. Don't be fooled into thinking that there is only a single serving in a package that may have two, three, or even five servings. Figure 14.2 below shows a bag of chips with 18 portions, more than 2500 calories, and 360 carbs.

5. When All Else Fails, Use Your Hand to Measure

The hand method ensures that you are eating portions relative to your body size. Because the meal is based on the hand size, men will more likely be eating a larger share than women. Children with tiny hands need even smaller portions. While this method is only an

Figure 14.2 *Large Bag of Chips with 18 Portions and 2340 Calories*

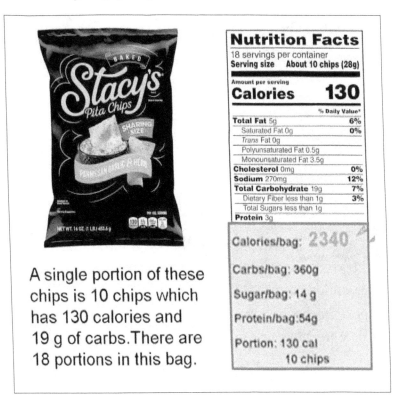

approximation (nothing can be as accurate as a scale), it helps keep portions at a reasonable size and serves as a good gauge for how much to eat when away from home. Figure 14.3 illustrates using your hand to estimate food portions.

The following are tips to help you:

- A serving of protein should be about the size of the palm of your hand.
- Eat a salad that is the size of both hands put together.
- Green vegetables should be the size of about two fists.
- Starchy items like potatoes or pasta should be served in a portion about the size of one tightly clenched fist.

Figure 14.3 *Portion Size Using Your Hand*

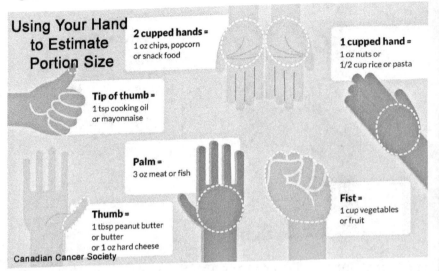

Using Your Hand to Estimate Portion Size

2 cupped hands = 1 oz chips, popcorn or snack food

1 cupped hand = 1 oz nuts or 1/2 cup rice or pasta

Tip of thumb = 1 tsp cooking oil or mayonnaise

Palm = 3 oz meat or fish

Thumb = 1 tbsp peanut butter or butter or 1 oz hard cheese

Fist = 1 cup vegetables or fruit

Canadian Cancer Society

Semaglutides taken in the appropriate dose for the individual makes portion choices easy. Small portions seem like large portions in that they are filling and stay filling for hours. The average dieter is accustomed to the often used combination of small portions, hunger and feelings of deprivation to lose weight. This is seldom observed in people taking the Semaglutides.

CHAPTER 15

Slow Weight Loss on Semaglutides

Given the novel chemical methods by which Semaglutides work in the body, its been found that certain behaviors tend to enhance the working of Semaglutides, whereas other behaviors can retard the effects leading to slow or minimal weight loss. While some of these behaviors are surprising, many of them can be avoided. Figure 15.1 shows some of the usual and some unusual causes of slow weight loss

Figure 15.1 *Unusual Causes of Slow Weight Loss with Semaglutides*

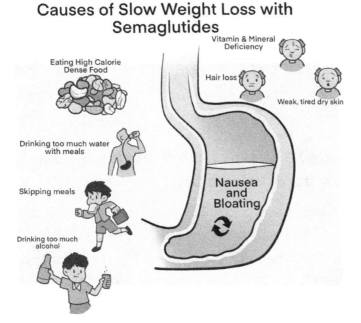

while on a Semaglutide weight loss program. Slowdowns after 8-10 weeks are often due to the usual slow downs in metabolism seen with all weight loss programs.

Drinking Excess Water May Increase Gastric Emptying

Sip liquids between meals, not with meals. Avoid drinking 30 minutes before a meal and wait about 30 minutes after a meal to drink anything. Drinking too much water with your meal may promote quick gastric emptying. Occasionally, too much water quickly especially will cause pain, nausea and even vomiting. Figure 15.2 shows the water restriction around meals, especially the evening meal.

Figure 15.2 *Limiting Drinking Fluids During Meals*

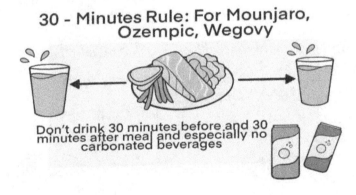

30 - Minutes Rule: For Mounjaro, Ozempic, Wegovy

Don't drink 30 minutes before and 30 minutes after meal and especially no carbonated beverages

Carbonated Beverages Accelerate Gastric Emptying and Slow Down Weight Loss

Carbonated beverages should be avoided. This includes beverages such as soda, beer, and sparkling water. When you drink carbonated beverages the carbon dioxide is released into your stomach. This occupies space in your stomach, causes it to expand, and create uncomfortable bloating symptoms. This results often in nausea, excess gas and acid reflux. In addition, the carbon dioxide occupies space in your stomach that could be taken up by nutrient-dense foods and liquids.

Many of these beverages are high in sugar and calories and leave the stomach fast without relieving hunger. Sugar, if present in many of these drinks is readily absorbed, raising blood sugar, and converting to fat. When the stomach has been emptied of food, it is filled with water and quickly empties causing more hunger. Some of the drinks to avoid include sparkling waters, zero calorie, no-sugar diet sodas (such as diet coke, coke zero, diet sprite, etc.), regular sodas and carbonated alcohol products as seen in figure 15.3. The problem with the common non-sugar, zero calorie "diet drinks" is they still are carbonated and may interfere with stomach fullness.

Figure 15.3 *Carbonated Beverages Speed Up Gastric Emptying Resulting in More Hunger*

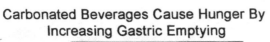

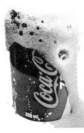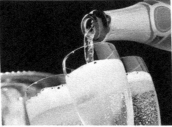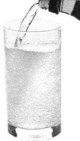

Injection of Semaglutides on Monday or Tuesday May Slow Weight Loss Down

Semaglutides are most effective in the first three days following injection, especially at lower dosages. Injecting early in the week, such as on Monday or Tuesday, lessens the control of hunger and cravings on Friday and Saturday since much of the drug has dissipated.

Injecting on Friday or Saturday morning maximizes the Semaglutide effects when they are most needed usually the weekend.

Dosage of Semaglutide is too Low

Everyone has a different reaction and tolerance to these medications. While low dosing is ideal to start treatment, some people simply need higher doses.

Sweet and Fatty Foods are Unpleasant to People Taking Semaglutides

Most people who take the medication dislike sugary and greasy foods. So why not simply avoid these. Sugary foods, white bread, pasta, rice, potatoes, granola, seeds, and nuts are not retained well in the stomach. High-carb foods will slow your weight loss; the carbs are quickly absorbed, raise blood sugar, and turn to fat. The stomach, emptied of the food, is then filled with water and quickly empties leading to more hunger and need for more food.

Avoid Large Meals, Skipping or Eating Too Fast

This is often the behavior that caused weight gain in the first place. Dieters need structure, eating times spaced throughout the day allowing time for breakfast, lunch, snack and dinner. After 3-4 weeks of taking any of these medications, the dieter often starts skipping meals because the medication produces fullness and lack of appetite especially during the day. The result is often a fall in blood sugar, fatigue and hunger leading to eating too fast or too much at dinner. This can result in nausea and even vomiting. *Instead of a single large meal, three to four little meals spread out throughout the day are advised.*

High Protein Shakes Should be Avoided

Just like water and carbonated beverages, high protein shakes tend to quickly pass through the stomach. A protein bar supplies the same calories, carbs and protein and would be a better choice.

Avoid Eating Dense, High Calorie Snacks

These food-like nuts, seeds, nut butters, and granola are very dense foods, high in calories, have difficulty with portion control and are not retained well in the stomach.

Eating Too Many Calories, Especially Carbohydrates

Often over looked after several months the slowing metabolism and boredom is often accompanied by the consumption of too many calories, especially carbohydrates. So faced with a slowing weight loss the dieter needs to reexamine how much is eaten.

Alcohol Causes Disinhibited Eating and has High, Empty Calories

Beverages like beer, cocktails and wine (especially white wine) are consumed often in large portions with subsequent large amounts of liquids. *In addition, many people underestimate the calories in alcoholic beverages.* One hundred calories per drink is a simple number to remember. Four or five alcoholic drinks a week might easily add 500-600 calories to each week's calorie consumption. In addition, alcohol makes weight reduction harder because it reduces metabolism, decreases food control, and often results in poor sleep.

A reduced desire or tolerance for alcohol has been reported by most of my patients taking Semaglutides. This becomes noticeable within a few weeks of starting the medication, often before the weight loss is obvious.

Vitamin and Mineral Deficiency

Deficiency in these essential nutrients can occur after large amounts of weight loss, especially if lost rapidly. This is often associated with numbness in the legs, especially at night, and thinning of hair. If you are losing more than 10 lbs. a month, I suggest a good multivitamin, potassium gluconate 595 mg a day, Magnesium 100 mg and Zinc 50 mg each three days a week.

Eating the Protein First

Most Americans will eat the salads and greens before the protein. However, in this plan you don't want to be so full that you cannot eat the protein part of the meal. If this becomes an issue, you may wish to switch to eating the protein first, followed by the salads and greens, European style.

Simple Changes in Semaglutide Plan Can Speed Up Weight Loss.

In addition to adopting some of the previously described modifications, the dieter can make a number of tweaks that can prevent plateaus and even accelerate weight loss:

1. Changing the injection day to Friday or Saturday as mentioned previously.
2. Splitting the weekly dose into two injections a week.
3. Adding small doses of appetite suppressors at the end of the week during periods of hunger.

MB is a 32-year-old medical doctor who I saw a few months ago. He had tried numerous diet programs. One of his worst problems was the 7-8 cans of Coca-Cola he drank every day. He weighed 320 lb. and called me after taking Mounjaro for a month proudly stating he has lost 6 lb. I told him he should have lost a lot more weight, maybe 15-18 lbs. during his first month. His response was that he was still drinking 7 sodas a day, but they were all diet coke. On further questioning, he stated that the diet cokes all day actually made him hangry. He would feel full for 30 minutes and after an hour or two, hungrier. I thought maybe he just kept emptying his stomach with each beverage.

RB is a long standing patient of mine who has tried repeatedly to lose weight. Despite multiple medications including many appetite suppressors and fat blockers he repeatedly lost and regained the weight. The major problem was inability to stop drinking 2-3 alcohol drinks a day. Some weeks it would total 21 to 30 drinks a week. When I told him that simply taking the Semaglutide injection would stop his interest and desire to drink, he could not believe it. As he recently said, "It's still unreal to me that most weeks I drink exactly one drink a week, which is the specialty drink we have with our London friends on our once a week teleconference. And in my case, since we try a different new drink each week, I keep buying new kinds of booze, and my dining room cabinets are completely overflowing with booze bottles, most of which have one or two servings removed, because after that one drink they just sit there. I'll even think during the week, well, I should use some of these boozes to make myself a new drink, and the right after ..is yeah, but I just don't feel like drinking alcohol."

CHAPTER 16

Weight Loss Slow Downs Due to Age, Activity, Medical Problems and Medications

Have a friend or family member that can eat a pint or more of Hagen Daz without gaining a pound while you gain weight after eating a spoonful or two? The answer lies in your metabolism—the energy consuming system that functions 24 hours a day. Metabolism is every metabolic process that is going on in your body. Each time you eat fat, protein, or carbs, the food is converted into energy that keeps all of your organs functioning. The faster the metabolism, the faster calories are consumed. The slower the metabolism, the more the calories can accumulate as stored fat. Metabolism is not simply a single number, but the sum of four processes going on at once as seen in figure 16.1. Some of the components of metabolism can be increased or decreased, while others are fixed.

Components of Daily Metabolism

A. **Basal metabolism: 1300-2000 calories/day.** This is the energy needed to breathe, maintain a normal body temperature, and maintain circulation and brain activity.
   Amount of Energy: variable but as much as 1300 to 2000 calories per day.

Can I Increase It? **NO**, it's fixed by genes, age, and gender.

B. **Digestion of food: 75-150 calories/day.** This is the energy needed to digest food.

Amount of energy: not much variation

Can I Increase it? **YES,** by selecting better food and drinks.

C. **Daily Activities: 150 to 300 calories/day** for people with sedentary jobs up to 1000 or more calories for people with strenuous jobs. (This is not the energy expenditure with planned exercise).

Amount of energy: extremely variable

Can I Increase it? **YES**, very easy to move around more, take stairs instead of elevator, park further from office or school.

D. **Planned Exercise: 0 to unlimited/day.** This is the traditional "exercise" component. It is not the exercise that occurs with activities of daily living, but the energy expended by walking or jogging around the neighborhood, playing sports, or going to the gym.

Figure 16.1 *Daily Metabolism Components*
Adapted from https://elizabethzrd.com/a-close-look-at-metabolism/

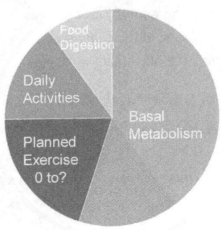

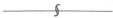
Factors That Affect Metabolism

- Age: Younger people have faster metabolism than older ones.

- Gender: Men have faster metabolism than women.

- Job activities: Many jobs simply are so sedentary they burn few calories.

- Medications: Numerous medications slow metabolism.

- Medical problems: Menopause, diabetes, hypertension, arthritis, and low thyroid function can alter metabolism.

- Depleted: vitamins, and minerals.

One of the overlooked secrets to weight loss, and especially weight maintenance is to discover the factors that may be slowing your metabolism and making a few simple changes.

Slowing Metabolism with Aging

Of all of the factors affecting daily metabolism, the most well-known one and least understood are the gradual slowing of metabolism seen with aging. There is a 2-3% drop in the basal metabolic rate every ten years. Usually at about age 35, most people start recognizing these changes. Table 16.1 shows decreasing metabolism with aging. Daily metabolism in women and men drops 270 and 282 calories per day respectively from age 20 to 70 for the same weight. This is the equivalent of walking about 3 miles or more a day.

New findings show the gradual loss of body cells, especially energy requiring muscle cells with aging. The result is a loss of five to six pounds of muscular tissue every 10 years starting in the late 20's. Add a reduction of physical activity and you have a simple formula for weight gain.

Table 16.1 *Basal Metabolic Rate Decreases with Aging*

BMR Related to Age

Age	Women	Men
20	1596	1798
40	1463	1648
50	1416	1597
60	1374	1556
70	1320	1516
Women: 160 lb, 64 inches		
Men: 195 lb, 70 inches		

Barry Stein of Wake Forest University School of Medicine explains: "As we age, we are subject to muscle wasting. Since muscle burns more energy than fat, this means the metabolic load goes down and metabolism reflects that. That is, if you do nothing your metabolism falls year after year."

There are things you can do to keep your metabolism effective. Exercise is No. 1. Exercise step-ups the amount and metabolic activity of mitochondria—the metabolism part of our body cells. This all suggests that elderly people may recover some of the resting metabolic rate by day-after-day anaerobic exercises.

Gender and Metabolism Differences

There are relatively small differences in metabolism between men and women. On average, women's total metabolism (the number of calories burned for basal metabolism—respiration, heart-beat, maintaining body temperature, digestion and exercises that occur with daily activities such as dressing, making a bed, taking the garbage out rather than planned exercise such as gym activities) is around 5 to 10 percent lower than men's. This is explained by differences in fat and muscle mass between the two sexes. Muscle mass and bones size are far larger in men than in women, even if though they are of equal weight. Women have a higher percentage of body fat (20-30%) than men (12 to 20%). For example:

A 30-year-old male weighing 160 lbs. has 72 lbs. of muscle and about 25 lbs. of bone and fat. A typical female of the same age who weighs only 125 lbs. has 38 lbs. of muscle, 15 lbs. of bone, and almost double the amount (30lbs.) of fat.

Because of these differences in muscle mass, a male simply burns up more calories at rest than a female.

Genetic Differences in Physical Activity

It is not as simple as built in genetic differences in resting metabolism between men and women. Every recent study finds that men are more physically active then women. Some of the differences can be explained by differences in job-related activities, while others are differences in intensity of extra exercise, such as gym activities and outdoor sports.

Since men burn more calories even when they are resting and more when they are moving about, women have greater difficulty losing weight than men. While gender differences in metabolism do exist, the differences in terms of total weight loss are small. For both men and women, making positive lifestyle changes is still the most important determinant of body weight, lifespan, and fitness.

Medical Disorders and Slow Metabolism

Thyroid disorder: Only disorders of the thyroid—hypothyroidism (underactive thyroid gland) and hyperthyroidism (overactive thyroid gland)—can actually slow down or speed up metabolism. Only 4% of the US population have an underactive thyroid gland, while less than 0.3% of the population have an overactive thyroid gland.

The incidence of hypothyroidism is much lower than one might expect from all of the attention given to it as a cause of obesity. In fact, the major problem is difficulty losing weight rather than as a cause of weight gain and obesity itself.

Low levels of thyroid hormone do cause bodily functions to slow down. The voice becomes hoarse and the speech slow, eyelids droop and the eyes and face become puffy and swollen. Minor weight gain, constipation and cold intolerance are common. The hair becomes sparse, coarse, dry, scaly, and thick. Some older people may appear confused, forgetful, or demented—signs that can easily be mistaken for Alzheimer's Disease or other forms of dementia. Figure 16.2 shows the typical signs and symptoms of low thyroid.

Figure 16.2 *Signs of Hypothyroidism*

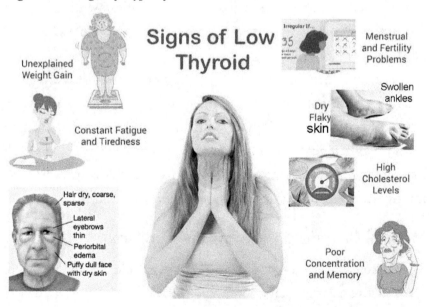

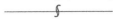
Type 2 Diabetes: Another cause of slowdown of metabolic activities is type 2 diabetes. It is not completely clear why diabetics have slow metabolisms, but they seem to have more trouble taking off weight than non-diabetics. This may be related to their higher blood sugar levels which fools the body into believing there is lots of energy around, resulting in a slowdown in metabolism.

Medications and Slow Metabolism

Struggling to lose weight and not getting anywhere? Maybe gaining weight on medications? Are your prescription medications slowing down your weight loss?

Steroids, Estrogens, Diabetic and Blood Pressure Drugs

While no one knows exactly how many prescription drugs can cause weight gain, experts estimate the list includes more than fifty common medications, the most common being steroids, estrogens, and anti-depressants. The medication-associated weight gain can be a few pounds—or as much as thirty pounds over several months.

The anti-seizure medication Depakote, diabetes drugs like glyburide and Januvia, and the high blood pressure drugs Cardura and Inderal cause drug-induced weight gain. Heartburn drugs like Nexium and Prevacid may also cause drug-induced weight gain.

Psycho-active Drugs Lead the Way in Weight Gain

Older mono-amine oxidase inhibitors like Parnate and Nardil as well as anti-psychotic medications, Olanzapine and Clozapine have been associated with very significant weight gain. The SSRI group of antidepressants including Paxil, Zolofot and Effexor also produce weight gain but to a lesser degree. Paxil may have the greatest weight gain from this group.

It is not possible to predict who's most likely to gain weight from taking antidepressants. However, recent research has shown that people who gain weight within the first few weeks more commonly have weight problems later on during the treatment.

Overall, it's estimated that the chance of gaining significant weight with anti-depressants is about 25%. That is a very large number and needs to be considered carefully. One of the first things I do with a new patient struggling to lose weight is to review the medications, especially the prescription ones, and the dose levels.

What to do if You Suspect Your other Medications May Play a Role in Difficult Weight Loss

As indicated, medication most involved in weight gain or failure to lose weight include the psychoactive, diabetic and hypertension drugs. If suspected, never stop them suddenly without a plan. That may be even worse. Keeping in mind that everyone responds to these drugs differently, switching to a different but similar medication can often lessen the weight problems. Paxil has the most problems among the Selective Serotonin Reuptake Inhibitors (SSRIs) while Celexia has the least. Recent evidence suggesting adding small doses of seizure drugs such as Topamax, Metformin or a drug used for alcoholism, Naltrexone may lessen the problem.

After rapid weight loss, as seen with these medications, it's possible to experience vitamin and mineral deficiencies. It's easy to add vitamins and minerals such as potassium, magnesium and zinc.

CHAPTER 17

Exercise, Metabolism and Weight Loss

The weight maintenance equation is the balance between the calories we consume through eating and drinking and the calories we burn through non-exercise thermogenesis (breathing, digestion, heart rate, etc.) and actual exercise; whether as part of daily life or as part of an activity program.

The phrase 'physical activity' and the word 'exercise' are used interchangeably. When properly defined, physical activity is any motion that results in energy expenditure, whereas exercise is planned, regulated physical activity.

The American Diabetes Association (ADA), the American Academy of Clinical Endocrinologists (AACE), and the National Academy of Nutrition and Dietetics all promote exercise as a vital component of any weight management program. Exercise is linked to improved cardiovascular fitness, insulin sensitivity, type 2 diabetes management, blood sugar management, blood pressure regulation, and, in some cases, depression.

Important Exercise and Weight Loss Questions

1. Is exercise necessary for weight reduction and weight maintenance?

2. Which comes first, food restriction or exercise?

3. Is aerobic and resistance exercise different in weight loss or maintenance?

4. How important is exercise in maintaining weight after weight loss?

5. What are the reasons for less weight reduction with exercise than predicted?

6. How does psychological effect of exercise benefit weight loss?

Is Exercise Necessary for Weight Loss and Weight Maintenance?

Most, but not all studies show that exercise alone has a negligible impact on weight loss. The American Academy of Sports Medicine and the American Diabetes Association declare in a joint policy statement that "when relying solely on exercise for weight loss, up to 60 minutes per day or more may be necessary." Even with this level, the weight loss in the exercise groups was no greater than 2-3 lbs. in 3 months as compared to the non-exercise group.

The American College of Endocrinology in 2016 recommended "aerobic training of 150 minutes per week." Even with this high duration, vigorous exercise in very committed individuals was only able to produce a weight loss of 3-4 lbs after a year.

This research implies that for the ordinary person who has difficulty completing any exercise on a regular basis, "60 minutes of exercise a day or even 150 minutes a week" simply will not happen for the average American on a regular or nearly permanent basis. More importantly, even if achieved, it does not result in a significantly larger weight reduction than calorie restriction alone.

Caloric-Restricted Diet or High-Intensity Exercise?

In a randomized, controlled trial of 52 obese men, Ross et al. found that the exercise-only group lost the same amount of weight as the calorie restriction group over three months (16 lbs.). Based on the aim of a daily 700-calorie energy expenditure (60 minutes per day), it may be necessary to exercise for longer than the minimum national recommendations of 150 minutes per week in order to achieve clinically significant weight reduction.

Aerobic Training vs. Resistance Training for Weight Loss

Aerobic exercise (calorie equivalent to twelve miles/week), resistance exercise (3 days/week), and a combination of the two were compared without change in food intake over eight months. Aerobic exercise resulted in more weight loss and fat mass decrease than strength training. (3.8 lb. vs. 1.8 lbs. for the aerobic and resistance groups, respectively)

Role of Exercise in Weight Loss Maintenance

Physical exercise plays an important role in weight management after losing weight, but the level of exercise alone required may be beyond the capability and personal preferences of most weight losers. In the National Weight Control Registry (NWCR), 90% of individuals reported exercising to maintain long-term weight reduction, with an average of *383-calorie expenditure* seven days per week. However, 383 calories of exercise daily may be too much for many individuals to continue on a regular daily basis. Other studies have found that even greater levels of physical activity are needed. This includes Tate et al. who observed those who exercised more than 2,500 calories per week gained less than half the weight as those who exercised less than 2,500 calories per week.

What is the Reason for Less Weight Loss than Predicted?

Despite the fact that everyone's metabolism and calorie-burning capacity vary widely, researchers determined that only around 71% of calorie expenditure through exercise and general activity is translated into higher caloric expenditure for that day. Our bodies "compensate" for the increased level of physical activity by reducing their resting basal energy expenditure following the exercise resulting in fewer calories being expended.

Aerobic Exercise More Important than Resistance Training

Aerobic exercise directly increases your metabolism. Aerobic activities like walking or running burn more calories than strength-building activities like weightlifting. But it is important to note that muscle burns calories, while fat does not. This means that the more muscular you are, the higher your metabolism will always remain. It's often a delicate balance between choosing aerobic vs. resistance training. Figure 17.1 shows how varied aerobic exercise can be.

Keep Yourself in Motion Regularly

After regular exercise such as walking, biking and swimming, your metabolism rate will increase not only during the activity but for several hours after.

Weightlifting: The More You Increase Your Muscle Mass the More Your Metabolism Will Increase

Most lay articles and trainers overestimate the effect of muscle on metabolism. The best estimate is that muscle contributes an

Figure 17.1 *Varieties of Aerobic Exercises*

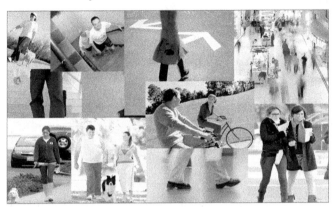

average of 6 kcal/lb. Muscle contributes about 20% to the day's total metabolism. It's interesting to note that the combined metabolism of the heart, kidneys, lungs, brain, and liver are 80% of the day's metabolism, far greater than muscles.

What is the Effect of Increasing Muscle Mass on Daily Metabolism?

Not as much as you might think. Most peer-reviewed resistance studies in humans reported an increase of only 2.2 to 4.5 lbs. of muscle mass! Not what you hear in the gym. This would increase the metabolic rate by about 50 calories per day at best!

Perhaps the real value of building muscle mass is that it helps prevent the loss of fat-free mass. Therefore, the additional muscle you build up, the greater you're resting metabolic rate (RMR). Every muscle fiber that you acquire perpetually burns up calories for you, even while you rest, and increases even more when you exercise. This is the only way to truly increase your metabolism permanently.

Don't think you have time to go to the gym? You will be able to increase metabolisms with only two 12-minute weightlifting sessions per week. This means that the more muscular you are, the higher your metabolism will remain at all times. After regular exercise such as walking, biking and swimming, your metabolism rate will increase not only during the activity but for several hours after.

Exercise Contributes Psychological Benefits for Weight Loss

Exercise has long been known for its physical benefits, but its psychological effects are equally crucial in achieving successful weight loss. The mind-body connection plays a vital role in shedding those extra pounds, making exercise a potent tool to tap into this synergy.

Firstly, exercise *enhances mood and reduces stress.* Physical activity triggers the release of endorphins, the brain's "feel-good" chemicals, which alleviate feelings of anxiety and depression helping individuals to maintain a balanced diet and stay on track with their weight loss goals.

Secondly, exercise *boosts self-confidence and self-esteem.* As individuals see progress in their physical abilities and appearance, they gain confidence in their ability to achieve their weight loss targets. Thirdly, exercise *improves cognitive function.* Regular physical activity has been shown to enhance mental clarity and decision-making skills. With increased mental acuity, individuals can make better choices concerning their dietary habits and overcome temptations that could hinder their weight loss journey.

Moreover, exercise helps *combat emotional eating.* By channeling negative emotions or stress into physical activity, individuals are less likely to turn to food for comfort, which is often a significant barrier to weight loss success.

In summary, the psychological effects of exercise play a critical role in achieving weight loss goals. By improving mood, self-confidence, cognitive function, and emotional eating habits, exercise empowers individuals to overcome mental hurdles and stay committed to their weight loss journey.

CHAPTER 18

Why do the Majority of Dieters Regain Weight Once They Stop Dieting?

Losing weight can be a challenging journey, but what's even more disheartening is when the lost pounds come creeping back. Currently, one-third of Americans are obese, and more than 60% are on a diet at any time! Most of the individuals find it tough to lose weight, but maintaining weight loss is even more difficult even with the best of intentions. The majority of those who lose a significant amount of weight will gain it back within two to three years.

Weight Rebound is a Normal Biologic Process-not Weakness or Lack of Effort

Weight return after losing weight is the result of biology, not a lack of effort or plan adherence. The natural reaction of an individual who has made many attempts at weight loss only to regain the weight is to think that he is weak and incapable of losing weight, even though the weight regain is a normal process.

Dieting causes a number of physiological processes to prevent what the body thinks is a state of "starvation." This includes hormonal changes that increase appetite and decrease metabolism. Made worse is environmental influences that encourage eating.

Internal Forces Responsible for Weight Rebound:

A. Hormonal Changes that Regulate Appetite and Satiety

The body interprets weight loss as starvation and makes hormonal adaptations that increase appetite and decrease satiety (fullness) including:

1. Reduction in leptin (the hormone released from fat discouraging eating).
2. Increase in ghrelin (the hormone encouraging eating).
3. Decrease in peptide YY (the hormone released reducing appetite).
4. Decrease in GLP-1 (the active ingredient in all Semaglutides) and GIP (gastric inhibitory peptide, the second of the active ingredients in the tirzepatides). Reduction of GLP-1 and GIP levels encourages eating and eventual weight regain.

B. Slowing of Metabolism (Metabolic Adaptation)

Metabolic Adaptation is a process of gradual slowing of metabolism that contributes to weight gain. It is also called Adaptive Thermogenesis. It's not as important as the hormonal factors which may be four times as much.

These hormonal and metabolic changes explain the common observed pattern of early rapid weight loss that plateaus after several months, followed by slow but progressive weight regain.

In figure 18.1, a group of overweight and obese individuals participated in three different weight loss diets over a period of 48, 92 and 128 weeks. Following each diet, there was the expected fall in weight (red lines) followed by a rebound to a higher weight. The metabolic rate (blue line) fell during each diet attempt, and post diet returned to lower and lower levels. Following each diet attempt, the body weight post-diet (red lines) gradually rose to higher levels.

Figure 18.1 *Repeated Weight Loss Attempts and Weight Regains*
(Adapted from https://www.precisionnutrition.com/reverse-dieting)

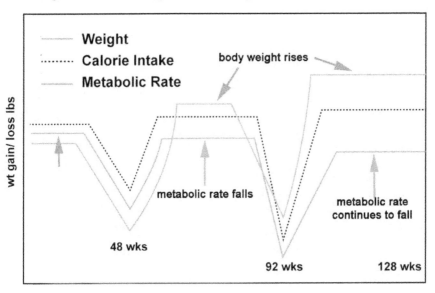

Weight Loss and Regain Following Three Different Diet Plans

How Can Most People Not Recognize That They Are Eating More?

Studies indicate that signals to the brain may be below the level of consciousness. As a result, the dieter is frequently unaware of the increase in appetite and food consumption; portions become larger, and food choices become higher in calories and carbohydrates. Making recognition of this problem even more difficult is the fact that they happen so slowly and relentlessly often over the years.

External Factors Responsible for Weight Rebound

1. Overconsumption of High Calorie, High Carb Food

High-density, highly-caloric foods which are inexpensive and easy to get results in mindless eating, bingeing, and night eating. Ultra-processed foods now contribute to the majority of foods eaten in the US. Fewer individuals make meals at home, and more people eat out or order take-out.

2. Limit in Physical Activity

Occupations are more sedentary, with more driving and less walking. The changes in food and physical activity drive people to increase their intake of food and decrease activity. The net is weight gain rather than weight loss.

3. Weight Loss from Exercise is Frequently Overestimated

The idea that exercising an hour a day and "burning" 3500 calories over a week, or reducing food intake by 500 calories a day for a week will result in a 1-pound loss of weight is mistaken. This calculation is incorrect because it fails to consider the reduced energy expenditure with substantial exercise.

When you alter one component, such as doing more exercise than usual or cutting the number of calories you eat in a day to lose weight, this sets off a cascade of changes in the body that affect how many calories you use up and, your body weight.

Weight Regain Occurs Following Weight Loss with Almost ALL Weight Loss Programs

Internal and external factors act together to produce weight regain after weight loss. This is observed whether the weight loss is accomplished by 1. Simple caloric reduction with increased exercise, by 2. Anti-obesity weight loss medications—both old and new—and even by 3. Semaglutides. This is discussed in three important studies:

1. Weight Regain after Diet Based on Lifestyle Changes Alone—NO Medications

This is the standard weight loss plan that has been in use for hundreds of years. Lifestyle modifications when done alone, regardless of the dietary or behavioral intervention employed, results in *3-8% weight loss* at the end of a year. As seen in figure 18.2, fifty overweight subjects were followed on a reduced calorie diet with daily exercise, but no medications. Weight loss reached a peak of 8.4% loss in 10 weeks. Without changes in food intake or activity, the subjects gradually regained weight resulting in a net loss of 6% at 62 weeks from baseline.

Figure 18.2 *Weight Loss and Regain after 62 Weeks on a Simple Weight Loss Program*

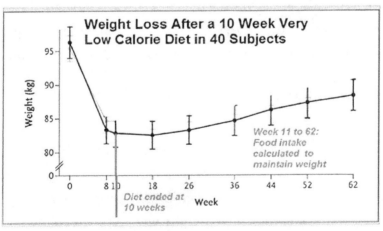

Adapted from Priya Sumuthran, Luke A. Prendergast, Elizabeth Delbridge, et al, The New England Journal of Medicine Massachusetts Medical Society Oct 27, 2011; https://www.nejm.org/doi/full/10.1056/nejmoa1105816

Numerous additional long-term weight loss studies with *no* medications involved demonstrate that despite sustained calorie restriction and increased activity, 70-80% of patients will return to their baseline weight by the fifth year following their weight loss.

2. Weight Regain after Diet Based on Lifestyle Changes and Anti-Obesity Medications (AOM, Excluding Semaglutides)

Seeking more significant weight loss and weight maintenance, AOM's that specifically address appetite and cravings have been utilized to support lifestyle changes but have been largely unsuccessful.

The average weight reductions on practically all pharmaceutical-based weight loss programs have been 10% or less at the end of a year. This is not substantially higher than when *no* medications are used.

Figure 18.3 shows 1590 subjects taking the weight loss drug Lorcaserin, a newer AOM medication. (It was taken off the marked several years ago because of other problems). It illustrates the concept that an AOM medication taken continuously over 2 years is inadequate to fully stop weight gain after a weight loss program. Note the weight gain of 4% over a year in the "Lorcaserin continued" group. In the Lorcaserin stopped group, there was a 10% weight gain.

Weight Regain after Diet Lifestyle Changes and Treatment with Semaglutides

In the STEP 1 Withdrawal Study treatment with Semaglutide resulted in 17.5% weight loss from baseline at the end of 68 weeks. At that time, the Semaglutide and lifestyle support were stopped. As figure 18.4 demonstrates weight was regained following the withdrawal (at 68 weeks) of the Semaglutide. After only 16 weeks on no therapy, half of the weight was regained. At 120 weeks (52

Figure 18.3 *Weight Regain after Loss with Anti-Obesity Medication Lorcaserin*

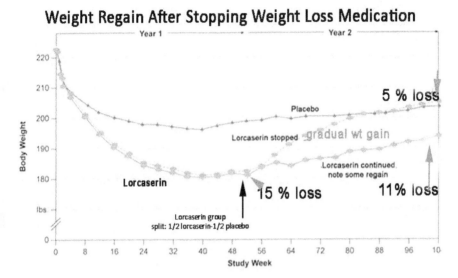

weeks with no treatment) the weight loss had fallen to only 5.6%. The study clearly shows that even with the most potent weight loss medication producing initially more than 18% weight loss, weight regain is a significant problem when stopping the medication.

Figure 18.4 *Weight Regain Following 68 Weeks of Semaglutide Therapy Followed by Withdrawal*
Adapted from Wilding, J. P. et al, https://dom-bs.onlinelibrary.wiley.com/doi/10.1111/dom.14725

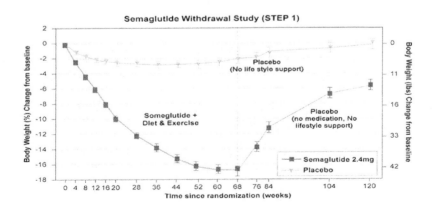

Weight Regain After Weight Loss Reverses Improvements in all Comorbidities of Obesity

As weight is regained, the improvements in comorbidities and other health problems disappear as the underlying problems resurface:

• *Metabolic Changes are First to Reappear:*

Blood pressure usually is the first function to rise, followed by blood sugar and cholesterol with weight regain. Medications for hypertension and diabetes that were discontinued have to be restarted. This whole process of weight rebound and return of metabolic problems is slow, subtle and often hard to recognize at first.

• *Physical Problems Return Last:*

As more weight is gained, patients complain of pain in their knees, back, and hips. A common complaint I see is pain walking up and down steps or some shortness of breath when rushing. Some patients notice the return of unusual fatigue during the day, an early sign of sleep apnea or acid reflux symptoms both due to increasing fat mass.

The weight regain associated with the return of major comorbidities of obesity necessitates the use of a new weight maintenance strategy, which is covered in the next chapter.

CHAPTER 19

Long-Term Semaglutide and Tirzepatide Therapy for Weight Loss Maintenance

Feelings of inadequacy and helplessness are often experienced by many overweight and obese people who struggle not only with weight loss but with weight regain often accompanied by serious medical complications. Often these individuals have been very successful in every aspect of their lives, except for losing and then maintaining their weight loss.

Not receiving much empathy from the medical profession, they often are told they lack willpower or are lazy. All of this occurs in a setting where powerful hormones are produced to not only prevent weight loss, but to encourage eating of especially high-carb, high-fat, and high-calorie foods.

Three studies were presented that showed that weight regain after weight loss is the norm. This occurs despite a strict food and exercise plan, weight loss medications and even after bariatric surgery. The degree of weight regain can vary from 20% in some studies to 80% of starting weight in others. In many people, the weight often returns to a higher level than before the weight loss program started. This is the consequence of multiple factors mostly due to widespread hormonal changes designed to prevent what the body interprets as starvation during and especially after weight loss.

Unfortunately, weight regain is accompanied by a slow reversal of many of the improvements in blood pressure, heart function, diabetes and arthritis accompanying the weight loss. Patients who lose weight and stop their high blood pressure medication, cholesterol pills or even pain pills for arthritis, often have to slowly restart them as their problems return.

Semaglutides including Ozempic, Wegovy, Zepbound and Mounjaro have shown promise not only for safe and fast weight loss, but for long term control of body weight. In this chapter I summarize the use of these drugs not only for weight loss but for long term weight maintenance. I divide the dosing into those obese or overweight individuals who are nondiabetic and to those with type2 diabetes.

Treatment Doses of Semaglutides for Non-Diabetics: Manufacturer's Dosing of Semaglutides for Weight Loss

The dosing schedule from the manufacturer starts with the initial dose and then increases every month to the maximal dose. This is limited only by the side effects The actual monthly weight loss is not a factor in the increase in dosing. Note that doses beyond 17 weeks can either be 2.0 or 2.4 mg per week for the Semaglutides and 12.5 or 15 mg per week of the Tirzepatides depending on the response.

Dr Lipman's Weight Loss Dosing Plan for Semaglutides

The treatment with the Semaglutides is reviewed in details in chapter 8. Every patient I have treated has a different response to the medication in terms of hunger and cravings control, weight loss, and adverse reactions. This is based on many factors some of which are obvious such as initial body weight, age, gender, physical activity levels and eating patterns. A small number of patients can lose weight with the lowest doses of 0.25 mg per week of Ozempic/Wegovy and 2.5 mg per week of Zepbound and Mounjaro. More weight can be lost taking a little higher, but still a low dose of 0.5 mg per week of Ozempic/Wegovy and 5.0 mg per week of Zepbound and Mounjaro. My plan only increases the dose above the initial dose if slow weight loss is experienced.

Table 19.1 *Initial Dose and Titration of Semaglutides: Ozempic/Wegovy and Mounjaro*

Titration of Weekly Doses of Semaglutides for Weight Loss				mg/week	
	wks: 1-4	wks:5-8	wks:9-12	wks: 13-16	wks: 17+
Ozempic/Wegovy	0.25	0.5	1	1.7	2.4
Mounjaro	2.5	5	7.5	10	12.5 15

Usual starting

High Doses

As indicated, I suggest stopping the dose titration at whatever dose produces sufficient weight loss with the least side effects. That becomes what I term the EFFECTIVE DOSE. Sometimes, it's the lowest, and sometimes the maximum dose. More likely, it's the middle doses. I let the patient decide whether to start at the very lowest doses or the more common 0.5 or 5.0 mg doses per week previously described.

Guidelines to Help Determine the Effective Dose

1. **"Days to Hunger:"** This is the number of days following the injection when the patient starts noticing a return of appetite and cravings. The goal is to aim for 5-6 days. If the patient has hunger by the 3rd or 4th day after injection, the dose is probably too low. If the patient can go a whole week (or often almost a whole week) before

experiencing cravings and hunger, that is probably the best dose. Many patients forget to take the 2nd weekly dose because of lack of hunger. That may indicate too high a dose.

2. "Lapses in Medications:" Sooner or later, there are naturally occurring lapses in the medication from several weeks to often a month or more due to cost or unavailability. I ask my patients to pay attention to hunger and cravings during these lapses.

Many patients maintain their weight and control of hunger and cravings for 2 or 3 weeks after the last injection. A minority are able to go a month between injections without the return of significant hunger, cravings or weight gain. This provides a reasonable estimate of the effect of the medication in controlling appetite and the frequency of injections as well as appropriate dosages. This of course does not apply to patients taking the medications for diabetes and control of blood sugar even if they are obese.

Reaching Goal Weight and Selecting Maintenance Doses of Semaglutides in Nondiabetics

After the STEP and SURMONT Studies (Chapter 6) revealed effective long term weight loss, control of appetite and cravings as well as a lack of significant side effects, I decided to offer the Semaglutide and Tirzepatide treatments to patients who had reached their weight loss goals. The questions were dose and frequency of injections.

1. Dosing Based on Prescribing Information Available Online or from the Product Insert: The suggested dosages are usually the highest doses. This usually means Ozempic/Wegovy 2.0 or 2.4 mg per week or Mounjaro 15 mg per week. One might reduce one step if side effects are a problem. The frequency of injections continues weekly.

2. Dr Lipman's Dosing Plan for Maintaining Weight Loss: I base the maintenance dose on the dose of Semaglutide needed to lose the weight and the presence or absence of side effects. This begins by taking the "effective" dose every two weeks instead of weekly. After 2 months (4 injections), it can be reduced to once every three or even every four weeks. The four week intervals are not very common. I suggest keeping the dose as low as possible to avoid side effects and reduce costs. The end point in reducing dosage intervals is the return of hunger, cravings and weight gain. An alternative method is to continue with weekly injections, but to slowly decrease the dosage using the same endpoint.

The advantages of utilizing modest dosages of these medications include fewer side effects, lower costs, and improved availability. The goals remain the same with either method: maintain weight loss within a few pounds while continuing to minimize obesity-related comorbidities.

Whatever approach is utilized, it must be done over a long period of time—months or years rather than weeks. About 40% of my patients have been able to maintain their weight loss on these low doses. Others required higher doses, but only a minority required the maximal dose of 15 mg per week of Tirzepatides or 2.4 mg per week of Ozempic/Wegovy. When reducing the dose many of my patients complain of increased hunger two to three weeks after the last injection. In some patients this has been associated with a two or three pound weight gain. This quickly disappears several days after taking the next injection.

Maintenance of Semaglutide Dosing in Overweight Diabetics

This maintenance plan described here does *not* apply to overweight diabetics where controlling blood glucose using A1C values may be more important than the weight loss. Many people with diabetes who have used insulin and other diabetic drugs are concerned that increasing doses of Semaglutide might produce hypoglycemia like their prior experiences with insulin.

As noted, these medicines, when taken alone without any other medications for diabetes, only "normalize" blood sugar". Hypoglycemia is rare in diabetics and non-diabetic individuals.

In general, in this group of Semaglutide and Tiriezepatide users, once the optimum weekly dose is identified by careful titration to reduce the gastrointestinal adverse effects and optimize A1C, that dose is continued weekly like any other once-a-week diabetic medicine.

Summary of Maintaining Weight Loss after Semaglutide Treatment

All of the four Semaglutide medications can result in substantial weight loss that is achieved quickly and safely, and is associated with an improvement or elimination of many or all of the comorbidities. Unfortunately, the data also shows the regaining of half or more of the lost weight during the year after the Semaglutides are terminated.

The long term data show that without some mechanisms, the many forces causing weight regain after significant weight loss are beyond the control of most individuals, and significant weight gain remains in the future, albeit, sometimes very slowly for most people. Several proposed treatment plans for the continued use of Semaglutides after reaching the goal weight have been presented.

Most obesity researchers have reached these similar conclusions:

1. No amount of willpower, exercise, or dietary modification can prevent most of dieters from regaining some or all their weight sooner or later.

2. A consistent eating plan, physical activity, and lifestyle habits may be required to get the greatest potential long-term results.

3. A post weight-loss diet low in carbohydrates, calories, and fat, with high-quality protein and at least three servings of vegetables and fruits daily is optimal. Sugars and processed carbs should be avoided. Juices, and sugar-sweetened beverages should be eliminated and alcohol should be consumed in moderation.

Hunger, Diet Medication, and the Future

The strategy outlined in this book is based on the understanding that hunger can manifest itself in various ways. The sensation of hunger and appetite do not always represent actual hunger. Many signals encourage you to eat, but just a few hormones work to help you stop.

There is no magic bullet—no medicine, no matter how potent, can counteract the tremendous impulses that drives some of us to eat. Aggressive intervention, such as the Semaglutides and other novel drugs, may be necessary to lose weight and keep it off now and in the future.

JS is a patient I have treated with many weight loss medications and plans in the past. The last attempt with intermittent fasting and the keto diet led to fast weight loss and then rapid regain as his hunger and cravings returned. We had no real plan to help him keep the weight from returning to his usual weight of 302 lb. Taking Mounjaro when it was first available in 2022, he was able to lose 82 lbs taking 15 mg of the drug weekly. When he reached his goal, I suggested he taper the injections as indicted previously. He decreased the dose to 15 mg every other week and maintained the weight loss for 3 months. Then because he had lost his job, he could not afford even taking two injections a month and he decided to take a single injection at the first of each month. This worked out fairly well for him as he described a return of hunger and craving during the last 10 days of each month. He said after a few months he learned to expect the hunger and especially a return of the carb cravings and would be more careful during that time. He was happy to tell me that a few days after his monthly injection all of the added weight would disappear and he was able to return to his previous control of his eating, especially his carbohydrate cravings. Maybe not the ideal plan, but it is working for JS.

About the Author

Richard L. Lipman M.D., a board-certified internist and endocrinologist has treated more than 40,000 individuals with weight and metabolic disorders in his office in Miami, Fl. A graduate of the University of Pittsburgh, he did his internal medicine training at the Universities of Pittsburgh and Miami. While in training and in the Air Force, Dr. Lipman authored 18 publications in metabolism. He has recently authored the following eight books on obesity.

100 Calorie Secret

Diet Buddies: A Weight Loss Plan for the Whole Family

New 800 Calorie HCG Diet

La Dieta HCG

Restaurants and Recipes on HCG Diet

Qsymia Weight Loss Plan

2 Day A Week Diet

Glossary of Medical Terms

Agonist: An agonist is a chemical that binds to a specific receptor of a cell and triggers a response by that cell. Agonists often mimic the action of a naturally occurring substance.

Food Noise: a colloquial term made popular by social networks that refers to obsessive or intrusive thoughts about food which can affect people's daily lives.

GLP-1: Glucagon-like peptide-1 (GLP-1) agonists (also known as GLP-1 receptor agonists, incretin mimetics, or GLP-1 analogs) represent a class of medications used to treat type 2 diabetes mellitus and obesity. Examples of drugs in this class include exenatide, lixisenatide, liraglutide, albiglutide, dulaglutide, and semaglutide.

GIP Peptide: Gastric inhibitory polypeptide or gastric inhibitory peptide also known as glucose-dependent insulinotropic polypeptide abbreviated as GIP, is an inhibiting hormone of the secretin family of hormones. Its main role is to stimulate insulin secretion.

Leptin and Ghrelin: *Leptin*, which is made in our fat cells and *Ghrelin*, which is produced in our stomach signal our appetite centers in opposite directions. Leptin tells our appetite centers that our fat cells are full and that there is *no* need to eat while Ghrelin tells our brain that there is an empty stomach and that we *need* to *eat*.

Neuron: A neuron is a cell within the nervous system that conducts electrical and chemical signals.

Neurotransmitter: This is a chemical substance that is produced and secreted by a neuron and then diffuses across a synapse to cause excitation or inhibition of another neuron. Acetylcholine, norepinephrine, dopamine, and serotonin are examples of neurotransmitters.

Peptide: Peptide is a short chain of amino acids (typically 2 to 50) linked by chemical bonds (called peptide bonds). A longer chain of linked amino acids (51 or more) is a polypeptide. The proteins manufactured inside cells are made from one or more polypeptides.

Placebo: This is an inactive substance used as a control in an experiment or test to determine the effectiveness of a medicinal drug. The chemical is inert and has no medicinal benefit. Any symptoms observed when taking the placebo are believed to be due to chance or suggestion of the treating individual.

Placebo-adjusted rate: the placebo-adjusted treatment effect is the difference between weight losses with pharmacotherapy and placebo It is provided from data in randomized clinical trials.

Prescribing Information, FDA-approved Prescribing Information (PI) or Package Insert: also known as United States Prescribing Information (USPI), reflects FDA's finding regarding the safety and effectiveness of the human prescription drug under the labeled conditions of use. The *Package Inserts* which are included with each FDA approved medication establish the standard use of the medications. Its availability, ease of use, contents, and legal weight make the PI the resource that should often be the starting point when initiating a search for drug information.

Receptor: This is a molecule usually found on the surface of a cell that receives chemical signals from outside the cell. Every cell in our body has different receptors; each one has a different function.

Satiation: Satiation is the feeling of fullness achieved during food consumption, which promotes the termination of eating during a meal. Gastric stretch receptors detect the distension of the stomach wall in the presence of food, which directly stimulates neuronal pathways to the brain to trigger fullness and appetite reduction.

Satiety: Satiety is the lack of appetite or hunger for a period following a meal. It is largely controlled by a combination of hormonal signals in response to food in the gastrointestinal tract and nutritional or physiological factors.

Serotonin: Serotonin is a chemical found all over the body. In the brain, it acts as a neurotransmitter to send messages between cells. Serotonin affects the brain centers involving sleep, sex, and feelings of well-being, appetite and cravings.

Serotonergic: Refers to medications whose mechanism of action is to increase serotonin levels in the brain.

Synapse: This is the area between neurons where chemical messages are carried from one neuron to another.

Titration of medication: Slowly raising and lowering dosage of medications is used by physicians to achieve the best clinical response is known as drug titration. Drug titration is a way for clinicians to personalize medication doses so that patients can obtain the intended benefits of the treatment of their disease while minimizing side effects.

References

Ahmad NN, Robinson S, Kennedy-Martin T, Poon JL, Kan H. Clinical outcomes associated with anti-obesity medications in real-world practice: a systematic literature review. Obes Rev. 2021;22(11):e13326. doi:10.1111/obr.1332623

Almandoz JP, Lingvay I, Morales J, Campos C. Switching Between Glucagon-Like Peptide-1 Receptor Agonists: Rationale and Practical Guidance. Clin Diabetes. 2020 Oct;38(4):390-402.

Anderson, J.W., Konz, E.C., Frederich, R.C., Wood, C.L. "Long-term weight loss maintenance: a meta-analysis of U.S. studies." *Am J Clin Nutr.* 2001; 74(5): 579-84.

Apovian CM, Aronne LJ, Bessesen DH, et al; Endocrine Society. Pharmacological management of obesity: an Endocrine Society clinical practice guideline.J Clin Endocrinol Metab. 2015;100(2):342-362. doi:10.1210/jc.2014-34157

Astrup, A. The Satiety Power of Protein Am J Clin Nutr. 2005;(82):1-2

Baltaci D, Kutlucan A, Turker Y, Yilmaz A, Karacam S, Deler H, Ucgun T, Kara IH. Association of vitamin B12 with obesity, overweight, insulin resistance and metabolic syndrome, and body fat composition; primary care-based study. Med Glas (Zenica). 2013 Aug;10(2):203-10.

Batterman, R.L., Heffreon, H., Kapoor, S., et al. Critical role of peptide YY in protein- mediated satiation and body weight regulation. Cell Metabolism. 2006; 4(2): 223-33.

Bays HE, Fitch A, Christensen S, Burridge K, Tondt J. Anti-obesity medications and investigational agents: an Obesity Medicine Association (OMA) Clinical Practice Statement (CPS) 2022.Obesity Pillars. 2022;2:100018. doi:10.1016/j.obpill.2022.1000189

Bays, H. E. Lorcaserin: drug profile and illustrative model of the regulatory challenges of weight loss drug development. Expert Rev. Cardiovas Ther 9(3), 2011;265-277.

Calderon G, Gonzalez-Izundegui D, Shan KL, et al. Effectiveness of anti-obesity medications approved for long-term use in a multidisciplinary weight management program: a multi-center clinical experience. Int J Obes (Lond).2022;46(3):555-563. doi:10.1038/s41366-021-01019-611

Caudwell P, Gibbons C, Hopkins M, et al.. The influence of physical activity on appetite control: an experimental system to understand the relationship between exercise-induced energy expenditure and energy intake. Proc Nutr Soc 2011;70:171–180

Costello T, Dorrell M, Kellams T, Kraska K. Review of pharmacologic weight loss medications in a patient-centered medical home. J Pharm Technol.2016;32(1):37-41. doi:10.1177/8755122515604858

Dagenais, G.R., Qilong, Y., Johannes, F.E. Prognostic impact of body weight abdominal obesity in women and men with cardiovascular disease. Am. Heart J. 2005; 149(1): 54-60.

Davies M, Færch L, Jeppesen OK, et al; STEP 2 Study Group. Semaglutide 2.4 mg once a week in adults with overweight or obesity, and type 2 diabetes (STEP 2): a randomised, double-blind, double-dummy, placebo-controlled, phase 3 trial. Lancet 2021;397(10278):971-984. doi:10.1016/S0140-6736(21)00213-0 22

Davies M, Pieber TR, Hartoft-Nielsen M, Hansen OKH, Jabbour S, Rosenstock J. Effect of Oral Semaglutide Compared With Placebo and Subcutaneous Semaglutide on Glycemic Control in Patients With Type 2 Diabetes: A Randomized Clinical Trial. *JAMA.* 2017;318(15):1460–1470. doi:10.1001/jama.2017.14752

DeSantis, M. E., Korner, J., Leibel, R. L. Inhibition of Food Intake by Peptide YY3-36.N. Eng. J. Med.2003; 349: 2365-2366.

Diet Soda is Bad for You Bray, G.A., Nielsen, S.J., Popkin, B.M. Consumption of high-fructose corn syrup in beverages may play a role in the epidemic of obesity. Am J Clin Nutr. 2004; 79(4): 537-43.

Ello-Martin, J.A., Ledikwe, J.H., Rolls, B. "The influence of portion size and energy density on energy intake: implications for weight management." *Am J Clin Nutr.* 2005; 82(1): 236S-241S.

Flegal, K.M., Carroll, M.D., Ogden, C.L., Johnson, C.L. Prevalence and trends in obesity among U.S. Adults. 1999-2000. JAMA. 2002; 288: 1723-27.

Fletcher, A.E. Thin For Life: 10 Keys to Success from People Who Have Lost Weight and Kept it Off. Houghton Mifflin, New York, 2003.

Flier, J.S. Obesity Wars: Molecular progress confronts an expanding epidemic. *Cell.* 2004; 23: 337-50.

Flood, J.E., Roe, L.S., Rolls, B. "The effect of increased beverage portion size on energy intake at a meal." *J Am Diet Assoc.* 2006 Dec; 106(12): 1984-90

Fogelholm M, Kukkonen-Harjula K. Does physical activity prevent weight gain: a systematic review. Obes Rev 2000;1:95–111

Geier, A.B., Rozin, P., Doris, G. "A new heuristic that helps explain the effect of portion size on food intake." *Psych Sci.* 2006; 17(6): 532-5.

Ghusn W, De la Rosa A, Sacoto D, et al. Weight Loss Outcomes Associated With Semaglutide Treatment for Patients With Overweight or Obesity. *JAMA Net Open.* 2022;5(9):e2231982. doi:10.1001/jamanetworkopen.2022.31982

Gorgojo-Martínez JJ, Basagoiti-Carreño B, Sanz-Velasco A, Serrano-Moreno C, Almodóvar-Ruiz F. Effectiveness and tolerability of orlistat and liraglutide in patients with obesity in a real-world setting: the XENSOR Study. Int J Clin Pract . 2019;73(11):e13399. doi:10.1111/ijcp.1339925

Grundy S.M., et al. Definition of Metabolic Syndrome: Report of the National Heart, Lung and Blood Institute/American Heart Association Conference on Scientific Issues Related to Definition Circulation. 2004; 109: 433-8.

Haidari F, Mohammadshahi M, Zarei M, Haghighizadeh MH, Mirzaee F. The Effect of Pyridoxine Hydrochloride Supplementation on Leptin, Adiponectin, Glycemic Indices, and Anthropometric Indices in Obese and Overweight Women. Clin Nutr Res. 2021 Jul 22;10(3):230-242.

Hedley, A.A., Ogden, C.L., Johnson, C.L., Carroll, M.D., Curtin, LR., Flegal, K.M. Prevalence of overweight and obesity among U.S. children, adolescents and adults: 1999-2002. *JAMA.* 2004; 291: 2847-50.

Hill, J. O., Peters, J.C., Jortber, B. *The Step Diet Book*. Workman Publishing, New York, 2004.

Hill, J.O. "Preventing excessive weight gain." *Obes Res*. 2005; 13: 1302-3.

Hill, J.O., Peters, J. "Environmental contributions to the obesity epidemic." *Science*. 2003; 280(5368): 1372-74.

Houtkooper RH, Schrauwen P. NAD$^+$ metabolism as a target for metabolic health: have we found the silver bullet? Diabetologia. 2019 Jun;62(6):888-899. https://www.fda.gov/news-events/press-announcements/fda-approves-new-drug-treatment-chronic-weight-management-first-2014

JAMA Network Open |Nutrition, Obesity, and Exercise Weight Loss Outcomes and Semaglutide Treatment for Patients With Overweight or Obesity. JAMA Network Open.2022;5(9):e2231982. doi:10.1001/jamanetworkopen.2022.31982. https://jamanetwork.com/ on 04/19/2023

Janssen, I., Katzmarzyk. P.T., et al. Waist circumference and not body mass index explains obesity-related health risk. Am J Clin Nutr. 2004; 79: 379-84.

Jenkin D. J., Wolever, T. M. Glycemic index of foods: a physiological basis for carbohydrate exchange Am. J Clin Nutr. 1981; (34): 362-366.

Jastreboff, Ania M. et al, Triple–Hormone-Receptor Agonist Retatrutide for Obesity A Phase 2 Trial Https://www.nejm.org/doi/10.1056/NEJMoa2301972

Kershaw, E.E., Flier, J.S. Adipose tissue as an endocrine organ. J Clin Endo Metab. 2004; 89(6): 2549-56.

Klein S, Wadden T, Sugerman HJ. AGA technical review on obesity. Gastroenterology. 2002;123(3):882-932.doi:10.1053/gast.2002.3551418

Klem M, Wing R, McGuire M, et al.. A descriptive study of individuals successful at long-term maintenance of substantial weight loss. Am J Clin Nutr 1997;66:239–246

Korner, J., Leivel, R.L. To Eat or Not to Eat—How the Gut Talks to the Brain. N. Eng. J. Med. 2003(349): 926-928.

Kushner RF, Calanna S, Davies M, et al. Semaglutide 2.4 mg for the treatment of obesity: key elements of the STEP trials 1 to 5.Obesity (Silver Spring). 2020;28(6):1050-1061. doi:10.1002/oby.2279417

Lam, DD., et al, Serotonin 5-HT2c Receptor Agonist Promotes Hypophagia via Downstream Activation of Melanocortin 4 Receptors. Http://endo.endojournals.org/content/149/3/1323.abstract.

Lipman, R.L. The healthy aura: is eating low fat, lite, low carb or healthy food preventing Americans from losing weight? Am J. Bariatric Med. 2007; 22(1):18-26.

Lorcaserin: A Review of its Use in Chronic Weight Management. http://link.springer.com/articles/10.1007/s40265-013-0035-1

Mehta A, Marso SP, Neeland IJ. Liraglutide for weight management: a critical review of the evidence. Obes SciPract. 2017;3(1):3-14. doi:10.1002/osp4.8410

Metropolitan Life Insurance Company, New weight standards for men and women, Stat Bull159:40 1-4. Health statistics: http://www.cdc.gov/nchs/fastats/overwt.htm

Miles KE, Kerr JL. Semaglutide for the treatment of type 2 diabetes mellitus. J Pharm Technol. 2018;34(6):281-289. doi:10.1177/8755122518790925 13

Moholdt T, Wisloff U, Lydersen S, Nauman J. Current physical activity guidelines for health are insufficient to mitigate long-term weight gain: more data in the fitness versus fatness debate (the HUNT study, Norway).

National Center for Health Statistics. "Prevalence of Overweight and Obesity Among Adults." United States, 2003-2004. www.cdc.gov/nchs

Nestle, M. Increasing portion size in American diets: more calories, more obesity J Am Diet Assoc. 2003; 103(1): 39-40.Nichols, D. E. and Nichols, C. D. Serotonin Receptors: Chem Rev 2008, 108: 1614-1641.Nielsen, S.J., Popkin, B.M. Patterns and trends in food portion size. JAMA. 2003; 289: 450-3.

Ogden, C., Carroll M.D., et al. Prevalance of Overweight and Obesity in the United States 1999-2004. JAMA 295(13) 2006:1549-55.

Pollan, M. *In Defense of Food*. Penguin Press, New York, 2008.

Rolls, B.J., Hetherington, M. et al. The specificity of satiety: the influence of foods of different macronutrient content on the development of satiety. Physiol Behav 1988;(43):145-53.

Rolls, B.J., Liane, S.R., et al. Increasing the portion size of a sandwich increases energy intake. *J Am Diet Assoc.* 2004; 104(3): 367-72.

Rolls, B.J., Morris, E.L., Roe, L.S. Portion size of food affects energy intake in normal-weight and overweight men and women. Am J Clin Nutr. 2002; 76(6): 1207-13.

Rubino D, Abrahamsson N, Davies M, et al; STEP 4 Investigators. Effect of continued weekly subcutaneous semaglutide vs placebo on weight loss maintenance in adults with overweight or obesity: the STEP 4 randomized clinical trial. JAMA. 2021;325(14):1414-1425. doi:10.1001/jama.2021.322420

Rubino DM, Greenway FL, Khalid U, et al; STEP 8 Investigators. Effect of weekly subcutaneous semaglutide vs daily liraglutide on body weight in adults with overweight or obesity without diabetes: the STEP 8 randomized clinical trial. JAMA. 2022;327(2):138-150. doi:10.1001/jama.2021.2361916

Samara, J.N., Nielson J., Popkin, B. M. Patterns and Trends in Food Portion Sizes, 1977-1998 JAMA. 2003;289:450-453.

Schoeller D, Shay K, Kushner R. How much physical activity is needed to minimize weight gain in previously obese women? Am J Clin Nutr 1997;66:551–556

Schwartz, J., Bryd-Bredbenner, C. Portion distortion: typical portion sizes selected by young adults. J Am Diet Assoc. 2006; 106(9): 1412-8.

Sorensen, L.B., Moller, P., Flint, A., et al. Effect of sensory perception of foods on appetite and food intake: a review of studies on humans. *Int J Obes Relat Metab Disord.* 2003; 27(10): 1152-66.

Srivastava G, Apovian CM. Current pharmacotherapy for obesity. Nat Rev Endocrinol. 2018;14(1):12-24. doi:10.1038/nrendo.2017.1228

Stroebeie, N., De Castro, J.M. Effect of ambiance on food intake and food choice. Nutrition. 2004; 20(8): 821-38.

Sun Y, Sun M, Liu B, Du Y, Rong S, Xu G, Snetselaar LG, Bao W. Inverse Association Between Serum Vitamin B12 Concentration and Obesity Among Adults in the United States. Front Endocrinol (Lausanne). 2019 Jun 27;10:414.

Swift D, Johannsen N, Lavie C, Earnest C, Church T. The role of exercise and physical activity in weight loss and maintenance. Prog Cardiovasc Dis 2014;56:441–447

Tate D, Jeffery R, Sherwood N, Wing R. Long-term weight losses associated with prescription of higher physical activity goals: are higher levels of physical activity protective against weight regain? Am J Clin Nutr 2007;85:954–1003

U.S. Food and Drug Administration. FDA approves new drug treatment for chronic weight management, first since 2014. June 4, 2021. Accessed May 2, 2022.https://www.fda.gov/news-events/press-announcements/fda-approves-new-drug-treatment-chronic-weight-management-first-2014 15

Vosoughi K, Atieh J, Khanna L, et al. Association of glucagon-like peptide 1 analogs and agonists administered for obesity with weight loss and adverse events: a systematic review and network meta-analysis. EClinicalMedicine. 2021;42:101213. doi:10.1016/j.eclinm.2021.10121326

Wadden TA, Bailey TS, Billings LK, et al; STEP 3 Investigators. Effect of subcutaneous semaglutide vs placebo as an adjunct to intensive behavioral therapy on body weight in adults with overweight or obesity: the STEP 3 randomized clinical trial. JAMA. 2021;325(14):1403-1413. doi:10.1001/jama.2021.183121

Wadden TA, Chao AM, Machineni S, et al, Tirzepatide after intensive lifestyle intervention in adults overweight or obesity: the Surmount-3 phase 3 Trial, Nature Medicine, published on line, https://doi.org/10.1038/s41591-023-02597-w

Wansink, B. Environmental factors that increase the food intake and consumption volume of unknowing consumers. Ann Rev Nutr. 2004; ;Wansink, B. *Mindless Eating*. Bantam Books, New York, 2007.

Wansink, B., Chandon, P. Meal size, not body size, explains errors in estimating the calorie content of meals. Ann Int Med. 2006; 145(5): 326-32.

Weigle D.S., Breem, P. A. A high-protein diet induces sustained reductions in appetite, ad libitum caloric intake and body despite compensatory changes in diurnal leptin and ghrelin concentrations Am J Clin Nutr 2005;(82):41-8.

Wharton S, Liu A, Pakseresht A, et al. Real-world clinical effectiveness of liraglutide 3.0 mg for weight management in Canada.Obesity (Silver Spring). 2019;27(6):917-924. doi:10.1002/oby.2246224

Wilding JPH, Batterham RL, Calanna S, et al; STEP 1 Study Group. Once-weekly semaglutide in adults with overweight or obesity. N Engl J Med. 2021;384(11):989-1002. doi:10.1056/NEJMoa203218319

Printed in the USA
CPSIA information can be obtained
at www.ICGtesting.com
CBHW071143140724
11574CB00016B/172

9 798223 838389